REFLEXOLOGY

A Patient's Guide

An introductory guide to reflexology, explaining how it has been developed, what it can be used for, and how the treatment works.

REFLEXOLOGY
A PATIENT'S GUIDE

by

Nicola M. Hall

THORSONS PUBLISHING GROUP
Wellingborough, Northamptonshire
·
Rochester, Vermont

First published 1986

© Nicolo M. Hall 1986

British Library Cataloguing in Publication Data

Hall, Nicola M.
Reflexology: a patient's guide
1. Reflexotherapy
I. Title
615.8'22   RM723.R43

ISBN 0-7225-1229-5

*Published by Thorsons Publishers Limited,
Wellingborough, Northamptonshire, NN8 2RQ England*

Printed in Great Britain by Cox & Wyman Ltd,
Reading, Berkshire

5 7 9 10 8 6

Contents

Acknowledgements

The author would like to thank Jim Howden for the artwork, Ken Stephenson for the photography and Mrs Audrey Wall, the subject of the photography.

Introduction

During the past five years the interest in 'alternative' medicine has grown tremendously, helped by the increased publicity which the various forms of 'alternative' medicine have received from the media. Therapies such as homoeopathy, osteopathy and acupuncture had previously been better known but numerous television and radio features and articles in newspapers and magazines have greatly helped in making people aware of the lesser known therapies, including reflexology. This media interest has obviously been of great encouragement to all practitioners in these fields but one slight drawback of the increased publicity is that features on the subjects are often rather light-hearted and fanciful, particularly in the case of reflexology where the method of treatment involves the massage of reflex points in the feet. It is quite understandable that people will joke about this subject but it would be a great pity, if in doing so, they missed the important value of such treatment. There is more to reflexology than just 'toe-tickling'! If applied by a trained, skilled practitioner, the results of reflexology can often be amazing.

As with most of the 'alternative' therapies, the approach to treatment requires a consideration of the person as a whole. This approach is somewhat different from that of conventional medicine where individual symptoms are treated. The patient visiting their doctor will usually consult him/her about one specific problem which will then be treated but will often not mention other problems which may appear minor to them at the time or may be forgotten but which may well be relevant to the immediate specific problem. It is quite possible for different symptoms to be related. By treating the person as a whole, the symptoms may be removed or alleviated through finding the cause of the problem and correcting this also.

Another advantage of the 'alternative' approach is that patients have more time in which to talk about themselves to the practitioner. Instead of the normal ten minute appointment which the general medical practitioner will offer, a consultation with an 'alternative' practitioner will last considerably longer. In the case of reflexology an appointment will last for about one hour. This allows a better understanding between patient and practitioner and also enables a more thorough appreciation of the patient and his/her problems. There will always be a need for the very necessary service provided by medical doctors but more people are turning to the forms of 'alternative' medicine for a more complete approach to their health and health problems. People are also becoming increasingly more reluctant to take various drugs prescribed for them, being wary of any possible side-effects which may occur.

At present, unfortunately, not many doctors are aware of the benefits of reflexology, largely due to their lack of knowledge of the subject and their inevitable scepticism of the method. In general, the response which most patients would receive from their doctor if they mentioned that they were considering trying reflexology treatment would be that provided it did not do them any harm then there was no reason why they should not try it, but he/she might well add that it probably would not do them much good! There are, however, a few doctors who have been known to refer their patients to a reflexology practitioner and encourage such treatment and it would be heartening to see an increase in this trend though this may well take many more years.

It is hoped that the following chapters will explain more thoroughly what can be expected if the decision to follow a course of reflexology treatment is taken. They outline the history of the method, how it works and when it can be helpful, and emphasize the great importance of the feet. As will be seen, every part of the foot corresponds to a part of the body, so enabling the whole body to be treated through the feet.

This is not strictly a self-help/self-treatment book, although details of the treatment procedure will be given. Reflexology is a method which people often feel they can apply to themselves with just a little knowledge of the subject, but the best results will be obtained when treatment is given by a trained practitioner. Having read through the following pages, it is hoped that your interest in the subject of reflexology will be enhanced and that you will then decide to experience the benefits which this simple but effective method can so often have.

Chapter 1

What is Reflexology?

Today reflexology refers to a method of treatment whereby reflex points in the feet are massaged in a particular way to bring about an effect in areas of the body quite distant from the feet. There are also similar reflex points to be found in the hands, which may also be used for treatment, but where possible it is preferable to work on the foot reflexes since the response is better. Reflexology is derived from what was originally known as 'zone therapy', a term which is sometimes still used. There is, however, a slight difference in the two methods as a study of the history of the method will show.

History of the Method

The origins of reflexology date back at least 5000 years when the Chinese were known to have practised a form of pressure therapy with a basis similar to that of acupuncture. The ancient Egyptians were also known to be using similar methods in about 3000 BC as illustrated from tomb drawings where the feet were being held and massaged in a particular way. One of the earliest books to be written on the subject of Zone Therapy was published in 1582 by two eminent European physicians called Dr Adamus and Dr A'tatis. Another book on the same subject was also published shortly after this in Leipzig by a Dr Bell and it is known that at this time many people in the middle European countries from the poor to the wealthy, including royalty, all used a form of pressure therapy. In more recent times there has been evidence that some of the Red Indian tribes and primitive tribes of Africa have been using a form of reflexology.

The first real advancement of zone therapy can, however, be attributed to an American physician and surgeon from Connecticut called Dr William H. Fitzgerald. In 1913, Dr Fitzgerald commenced his research into the method of healing which he termed zone therapy. At the time he was head of the Nose and Throat department of the St. Francis Hospital in Hartford and was well respected as a medical surgeon and physician. He had graduated from the University of Vermont, spent two and a half years at the Boston City Hospital and two years at the Central London Nose and Throat Hospital. Then for two years he was assistant to Professors Politzer and Otto Chiari in Vienna and it was probably during this time in Europe that his interest in zone therapy began. On his return to America he developed this interest and began to incorporate zone therapy into his practice. Dr Fitzgerald must be admired for his courage in pursuing this work since his fellow medical colleagues were understandably not too willing to accept his new ideas.

The Findings of Dr Fitzgerald

Dr Fitzgerald had initially been intrigued by the fact that at times he was able to carry out an operation on the nose and throat without the patient experiencing much pain, while at other times a similar operation on a different patient caused considerable pain. He found that in the cases where little pain was felt, the patient had been applying pressure on certain parts of the hand or that during the examination prior to the operation, he himself had applied pressure to certain areas and these pressures had inhibited pain in other areas. With time, Fitzgerald traced these locations and described how the body could be divided into ten longitudinal zones — five on each side of a median line through the body. Each zone related to one of the five digits on each side of the body, with zone one extending from the big toe up the entire body to the brain and down the arm to the thumb, zone two extending from the second toe up to the brain and down to the second finger, zone three extending from the third toe up to the brain and down to the

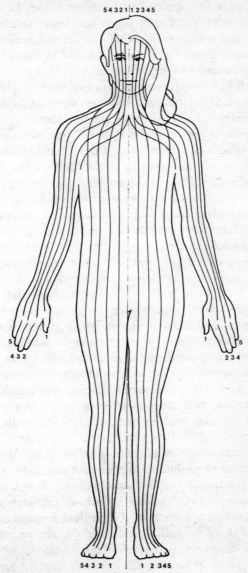

Figure 1.   The zones of the body.

third finger, zone four extending from the fourth toe up to the brain and down to the fourth finger and zone five, the outer zone, extending from the fifth toe up to the brain and down to the fifth or little finger. The description of the zones running from toe to brain and then down to the finger was not imperative and could have been described in the alternate way as running from finger to brain and then down to the toe. All of these zones extended right through the body from front to back and rather than being single lines, they were sections through the body of equal width. The zones did not cross in the head, as with nerves, so that the right side of the head and brain related to corresponding zones on the right side of the body and the left side of the head and brain related to corresponding zones on the left side of the body. By applying pressure to an area or areas in a certain zone, it was possible to inhibit pain in other areas within the same zone. (See Figure 1.)

Unknowingly, the basics of zone therapy are often applied by people as an automatic response to pain. People are known to grind or bite on their teeth when in pain and are, in fact, stimulating the zone areas which may well ease the pain. Likewise, a patient at the dentist's may tightly grasp the arms of the chair when undergoing treatment and this again is a way of applying pressure to the zones in the hand which may alleviate the pain being experienced in the mouth. Other automatic reactions to pain where pressure is applied can be seen in the person biting on their thumb after hurting it or the more obvious reaction of rubbing an injured and painful area directly.

The art of zone therapy initially involved the application of pressure to bony prominences throughout the body, especially the joints of the hands and feet and particularly the phalanges (bones of fingers and toes). The amount of pressure necessary to alleviate pain was such that it was firm enough to elicit a certain amount of bearable pain but not severe enough to damage any underlying tissues. The pressure, which was between 2 and 10 lb (1 and 4.5 kg), was applied for varying lengths of time but in general for between thirty seconds and five minutes, though sometimes more. Various constrictive gadgets were often used to apply a firmer constant pressure and it was not unusual for clothes-pegs or elastic bands to be applied to finger joints (see Figure 2) — this was accompanied by the warning that the constrictive articles be removed immediately should the fingers, toes or any another part of the body begin to show signs or appearance of blueness and it was recommended that the areas involved be massaged to restore the normal blood circulation! Pressure could also be applied using the thumbs or fingernails or a round-ended probe or end of a toothbrush. (See

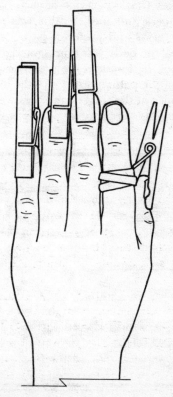

Figure 2.   The use of clothes-pegs and elastic bands on the fingers.

Figure 3.) Metal combs were also used, with the teeth of the comb pressing into the zone areas in the hands! (See Figure 4.) Although the hands were mainly used as the areas to which pressure was applied, rubber bands could be applied to other joints, including the toes, ankles, wrists, knees and elbows. Some practitioners also used electrical devices to stimulate the zone areas.

It became apparent as research progressed that, by applying pressure to the very ends of the fingers and toes, pain in any area of the corresponding zone could be eased. The anterior (front) and posterior (back) sections of each body zone met at the tips of the fingers and toes, so this was an area through which both the anterior and posterior parts could be reached. The anterior part of the body was represented on the back of the hand and the top of the foot and the posterior part of the body was represented on the palmar surface of the hand and the sole of the foot. The sides of the fingers and toes were also involved and related to the outer areas of each corresponding zone. In

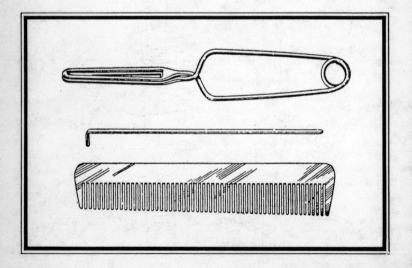

Figure 3.   Implements for applying pressure.

some instances it was found that when pressure was applied, the pain in the area being treated increased rather than lessened. This was later explained as an indication that infection or even a corn or callous existed in the area and so the cause of the problem had to be treated before pressure could alleviate the pain. This would involve possible removal of the corn or callous or treatment of the cause using pressure therapy but with the experience of more pain from the pressure until the condition was righted.

Dr Fitzgerald further described the existence of ten longitudinal zones within the tongue, again with five zones on either side of a median line. Pressure applied on the top of the tongue in the various zones affected the zones in the anterior part of the body. Pressure applied to the under surface of the tongue affected the zones in the posterior part of the body. For the tongue, pressure was normally applied using a form of metal probe though the fingers could be used too. One of the recommended treatments for hiccoughs was to wrap a

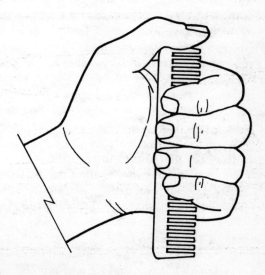

Figure 4. The use of a comb for applying pressure.

handkerchief around the fingers and then pull the tongue out as far as possible and grasp it firmly! The hard and soft palate could also be divided into ten zones, including the upper jaw. Pressure or contact on the posterior surface of the teeth and gums affected the posterior parts of the zones throughout the body and pressure to the anterior surfaces affected the anterior parts of the zones. Similarly, zones within the pharynx (the cavity at the back of the mouth) were such that the posterior surfaces affected the posterior parts of the zones and anterior surfaces affected the anterior parts of the zones. The anterior and posterior surfaces of the lips also related respectively to the anterior and posterior parts of the zones and the teeth could be treated by pressure to an area within the zone in which they were situated; for example, the incisors were represented in zone one and the molars in zones three and four. Another finding was that an infection in the pharynx or nose or mouth or even the vagina and rectum could be responsible for not only local irritation but also pathological changes in areas remote from the site of infection but traceable to the same zone.

Many examples of Dr Fitzgerald's work could be given and he particularly would give instances of treating headaches, eye problems, goitres, fibroids in the uterus, breast lumps and breathing problems — all responding well to his therapy. It was stated that pressure therapy was effective in 65 to 75 per cent of all the cases treated and this was a high success rate. When questioned on the validity of the method, Dr Fitzgerald often responded with a practical demonstration which was a more convincing way of answering his critics. One of his popular examples was to apply pressure to the specific part of the little finger which would then anaesthetize the ear, on the same side of the body. This then allowed him to place pins in the pinna (outside lobe) of the ear without any discomfort to the person.

Other Pioneers of the Method

The work of Dr Fitzgerald was first publicized by Dr Edwin F. Bowers who was a medical critic and writer from New York. He had visited Dr Fitzgerald and studied with him for a time before presenting articles on zone therapy in the press — it was, in fact, Dr Bowers who termed the method zone therapy. The medical world did not respond very favourably to this new method but more support was found from practitioners of natural medicine such as chiropractors, osteopaths and naturopaths. However, there was some interest from fellow doctors, some of whom researched further into the subject and made valuable contributions to the development of the method. These persons included Dr George Starr White, Dr Joe Riley and his wife Elizabeth Riley. Dr Riley wrote numerous books on the subject and also introduced the use of 'hook work'. 'Hook work' was so called because it involved the fingers of the practitioner being hooked over some part of the body of the patient in order to manipulate that area. The method could be used on the tissues, for example to lift a prolapsed womb, or on the joints such as the clavicle (the collarbone), the scapula (the shoulder blade), the ribs, the sternum (the breastbone), the iliac crests and pubic bones (parts of the pelvis) and the coccyx (the tailbone). All of these areas were thought to show five distinct zones, with the possible exception of the coccyx and the tip of the sternum which were thought to be able to affect the whole body if worked on and were therefore treated very gently. This 'hook work' could also be applied to bony areas within the same zone as the area needing treatment and in cases of, for example, an inflamed joint or nerve, a corresponding zone area could be worked on, such as the elbow for the knee or the shoulder for the hip.

Another great pioneer in the field was an American lady called Eunice D. Ingham who later become Mrs Stopfel after marrying one of her very satisfied patients! Having trained with Dr Riley, Eunice Ingham developed the 'Ingham Compression Method of Reflexology' and two books which she wrote called *Stories the Feet Can Tell* and *Stories the Feet Have Told* became standard textbooks for reflexology students. The Ingham method concentrated on the reflexes to be found in the feet and involved a special form of massage to reflex areas found on both the soles and tops of the feet as well as the foot digits. Eunice

Ingham had trained as a remedial therapist so had a para-medical background and she devoted herself in her later years to reflexology and the promotion of the method. In addition to a highly successful practice, she toured America extensively, lecturing, treating and training new practitioners.

The main pioneer of the work in Great Britain was a lady called Mrs Doreen E. Bayly who in her younger years had trained as a nurse. Mrs Bayly met Eunice Ingham while on a visit to her sister, a healer, in America. She was greatly impressed by the work and studied with Eunice Ingham before returning to England in the early part of the 1960s. After much perseverance, Mrs Bayly created more interest in reflexology in Britain and on the Continent and built up a busy practice as well as starting a training school for reflexology. Mrs Bayly deserves much credit for her endeavours to spread the interest in reflexology since initially there was very little enthusiasm for her work and substantial opposition, but gradually her efforts were rewarded. She died in 1979 just before her eightieth birthday at a time when reflexology was beginning to gain more acclaim. Her teachings are still continued through the Bayly School of Reflexology.

Reflexology has developed from the initial practice of zone therapy and in present times most practitioners of the method will concentrate on treating by massage to the reflex areas in the feet. The reflexes in the hands may also be used in some instances but generally those reflexes in the feet are considered more responsive. In a similar manner 'hook work' has been developed as an addition to foot massage and would be applied in a slightly less vigorous way than its original description by massaging joint or limb areas found in the same zones as the troubled areas; for instance, massage to the elbow for a knee problem or massage to the lower arm for a lower leg problem such as poor circulation. The use of gadgets for applying pressure is less evident and the thumbs or fingers are used to apply the required pressure in a more acceptable and more natural way of producing a healing response.

Chapter 2

How the Treatment Works

To many people, the idea of massaging the feet to improve their health seems too far-fetched to be taken seriously, but it is possible through reflexology treatment to help many disorders. As previously mentioned, in the feet and the hands there are reflex areas relating to all the parts of the body, so that the whole body may be treated through the feet. Every part of the foot corresponds to a part of the body, with reflex areas being found on the soles of the feet and also on the top and sides of the feet. The hands, likewise, contain reflex areas on the palms and backs of the hands.

The Zone Systems

The arrangement of the reflex points in the feet is such that they provide a logical map of the body; this organization of points is based on the zone system which exists in the body as described by Dr Fitzgerald. The ten longitudinal zones, as explained in Chapter 1, extend throughout the body with five zones on either side of a median or central line. These zones are not lines, such as the acupuncture meridian lines, but are sections through the body of equal width and extending from front to back. Whichever zone or zones of the body an organ exists in, there will be a corresponding reflex area in the same zone or zones of the feet. For example, the two kidneys are found in zones two and three on the right and left sides of the body, so reflex areas to the kidneys are found in both the right and left feet in zones two and three. Remembering that these zones do not cross in the brain, as does the nervous system, the right side

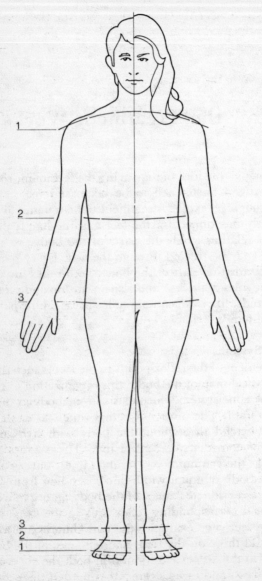

Figure 5. The transverse zones of the body.

of the body is represented in the right foot and the left side of the body is represented in the left foot, so the right kidney reflex is found in the right foot and the left kidney reflex is found in the left foot.

In addition to the ten longitudinal zones originally described, it has also been found that three transverse zones exist in the body which can also be described in the feet. These transverse zones can be seen in the body by drawing three imaginary lines as follows:

1. a line drawn across the upper shoulder girdle.
2. a line drawn across at waist level at the lower level of the ribs.
3. a line drawn across the level of the pelvic floor. (See Figure 5.)

The area above line one relates to the structures of the head and neck. The area between lines one and two relates to the structures of the thorax and upper abdomen. The area between lines two and three relates to the structures of the abdomen and pelvis. These areas can be transposed onto the feet and relate to the skeletal structure of the feet.

The Structure of the Foot

The feet are designed in a most clever manner and it is marvellous that such a relatively small area is able to support the human body with surprising ease even when the weight of the body may be somewhat excessive! The strength and mobility of the feet are achieved by the arrangement of the bones, muscles and ligaments of which they consist. Each foot is made up of twenty-six bones and in the feet are found one quarter of all of the bones of the body. Associated with the bones are nineteen muscles and one hundred and seven ligaments. Each foot has fourteen phalanges which are the bones of the toes, with each toe being made up of three bones except for the big toe which has just two bones. Leading back from the toes towards the heel are five bones called metatarsals with one relating to each toe. The remaining bones of the feet are called the tarsal bones with three cuneiform bones, a cuboid bone, a navicular bone, a talus bone and a calcaneum bone (the heelbone). (See Figure 6.)

From this bony structure of the foot, it is now possible to see

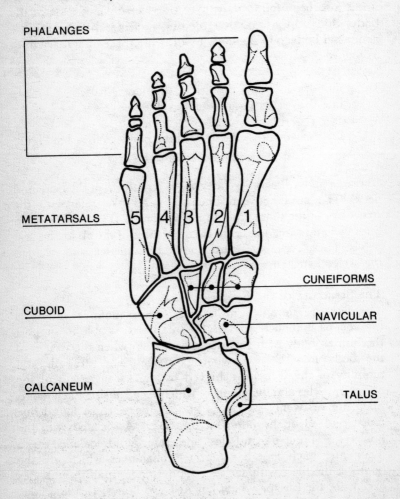

Figure 6.   The bones of the foot.

how the transverse zones of the body relate to the bones of the feet (see Figure 7):

Line 1 is at the base of the phalanges so that the reflexes of the head and neck are found in the toe areas.

Line 2 is at the base of the metatarsal bones so the reflexes of the thorax and upper abdomen are found in the area over the metatarsal bones.

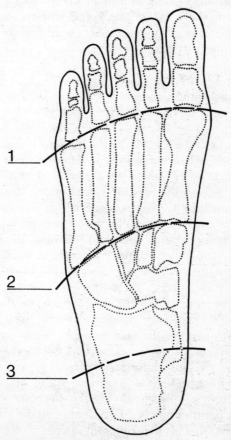

Figure 7. The transverse zones of the foot.

Line 3 is across the tarsal bones up to and including the ankle bones (inner and outer malleoli) so the reflexes to the abdomen and pelvis are found over the tarsal bones and around the ankle bones.

With the presence of both longitudinal and transverse zones in the body and the fact that these zones can be transposed onto the feet, there exists in the feet a 'grid-like' system which aids in the determination of the positions of the various reflex areas. There are a few slight exceptions to this pattern and these will be mentioned at a later stage, but for the majority of areas the zone pattern holds true.

How Does It Work?

Having established how the reflex areas can be described in the feet, the question then arises 'How does it work?' The exact reactions which take place when an area of the foot is massaged, resulting in an effect on a part of the body to which the area of the foot corresponds, are not fully understood. It is hoped that in years to come an explanation will be found; this would be of enormous benefit to the method since, understandably, some people are unwilling to accept ideas which cannot be proved scientifically even though results can be definitely seen.

Various theories have been put forward to explain the workings of reflexology and in very simple terms it is accepted that the treatment can have an effect on the blood circulation and the nervous system. A healthy circulation is vital for healthy functioning of all the body parts, with the blood transporting the necessary nutrients to the tissues and then carrying away from the tissues the waste products of metabolism. Reflexology can improve the circulation to all areas and thus aid this important transport system in the body to work to its fullest potential, in turn assisting the various body systems to function better. With the nervous system it is accepted that approximately 70 per cent of all disorders are due to 'nerve tension' in the different areas of the body and reflexology can be most effective in helping to reduce this tension, thus enabling the different areas to become more 'relaxed' and therefore function more efficiently. With many simple disorders the body is able to right itself without medication since it has a tremendous power to heal itself. Reflexology is able to help stimulate the healing forces present in the body and thus aid the body in its self-treatment.

Within the longitudinal zones described it is known that there is a flow of energy linking the organs within the same zone. The exact type of energy involved is not yet understood, though work is being done in this field in relation to the various forms of ancient Chinese medicine which work on energy systems. By the means of Kirlian photography, which is able to show the energy fields surrounding objects, it has been shown that the energy field or corona present around the reflex areas in the feet will be diminished when there is an imbalance in the body area corresponding to the reflex area. This corona will become improved or corrected, and therefore more defined, after reflexology treatment has been given, showing that the treatment has successfully balanced the energy field. The pain-reducing effect of reflexology may possibly be explained by the ability of massage of the reflex areas to cause the release of substances, known as endorphins, found in the brain which act as the body's natural pain-relieving agents.

Reflexes

The term reflexology is to some extent misleading. On hearing the term many people immediately think of reflex responses such as the 'knee jerk' when, by tapping just below the knee cap of the bent leg, the lower leg will extend and thus straighten — a reflex action. A reflex is, in fact, an involuntary response to a stimulus and many different kinds of reflexes have been described in the body. In most cases of these reflexes a reflex arc pattern exists with stimulation of a nerve ending (receptor), causing a nerve impulse to travel along a nerve fibre known as an afferent neurone to a reflex centre in the central nervous system, where a reaction occurs to send a nerve impulse along a nerve fibre known as an efferent neurone to the nerve ending (effector) in the part required to act. However, one type of nerve reflex arc, known as the autonomic reflex arc, differs from the simple reflex arc in that two efferent neurones exist, with the message passing from one to the other in an area (ganglion) outside the central nervous system. There are theories that claim that reflexology is working on this autonomic nerve pathway, though this is probably not the case. There are, however, in the feet 7200 nerve endings which interconnect through the spine and brain with all areas of the body.

When working on the various areas in the feet there may be some overlap with acupuncture points and areas connected with periosteal (bone) massage and lymphatic drainage techniques, but the reflexology areas are part of a separate and well-defined system requiring a specific form of massage. Whatever the correct scientific explanation for reflexology, and it may well be many years before the treatment can be fully explained, the fact that the method does work can be seen by the number of people who have received treatment and benefited from it — surely good enough evidence for many to justify trying it.

It is interesting that in a few cases practitioners have found that when working on areas of the feet, the patient has actually experienced a sensation in the body in the area to which the foot reflex area corresponded. This need not occur for the treatment to be effective, but occasionally patients do have this response. In one known case the patient actually experienced sensation in the body corresponding to every reflex point worked on — a very satisfying reassurance to the practitioner that the reflex areas are where they are reported to be!

Crystal Deposits
Another factor involved with the treatment is that in the feet, in certain reflex areas, crystal-like deposits may be felt by the practitioner. These crystals are presumed to be made up of calcium deposits which settle beneath the skin surface at the nerve endings in the feet. Approximately 1 per cent of the body's calcium level is present in the blood; this can readily be

deposited and appears to be done so more readily where there is tension present. The feet, in particular, are a site for these deposits since they are at an end point of circulation and the blood has to be circulated back up the leg against the force of gravity. These crystals feel to the practitioner like pieces of grit or gravel beneath the skin surface and by massaging these 'gritty' areas the crystals can be broken down and then be more easily removed by the blood circulation. Some authorities have stated that these crystals will always be felt in the feet when there is imbalance in the corresponding body area and that reflexology is all about dispersing the crystals. Although these crystals are often felt, it is not necessarily the case and reflex areas in the feet may indicate imbalances in the body without 'gritty' areas being present.

Balancing Effect
The work of reflexology is to balance up all the systems of the body and harmonize the entire body. The term 'out of balance' is used to imply that a particular area is not functioning efficiently either due to poor circulation to that area or tension in that area. Because the overall effect of the treatment is to balance, an overactive area will be calmed and an underactive area will be stimulated until the balance in the body is restored. The body is so easily thrown 'out of balance' by stress, diet or negative thoughts, and the resulting imbalances, even if only slight, will prevent 100 per cent efficiency of all the body functions. When working on the reflex areas in the feet, imbalances can be detected and by treating these areas the body can be brought back into balance and consequent better health.

Chapter 3

How the Treatment is Given

The first visit to somewhere new is frequently a slightly anxious experience for many people and especially when this also involves treatment of illness. Reflexology treatment is certainly not an unpleasant experience so should not provoke any additional anxieties! Often people are worried that the treatment is going to be very painful but again this should not be the case if the method is applied correctly.

Medical History
On the first visit to a practitioner, a detailed medical history of the new patient will be taken. This is helpful to the practitioner not only in assisting with the treatment procedure but also in making sure that no symptoms exist which would prevent treatment from being administered. Patients tend to remember the symptoms which are troubling them at the time of their visit but all symptoms and disorders experienced should be mentioned and for those with bad memories it is often a good idea to have written down a list of these before visiting a new practitioner! Any serious illnesses or operations will be enquired about and a patient should not feel embarrassed to mention any of these, however many, since they are all relevant to the complete health of that person.

Treatment Position
Once a medical history has been recorded, the patient will be asked to sit, ideally, in a recliner chair which will be tipped back

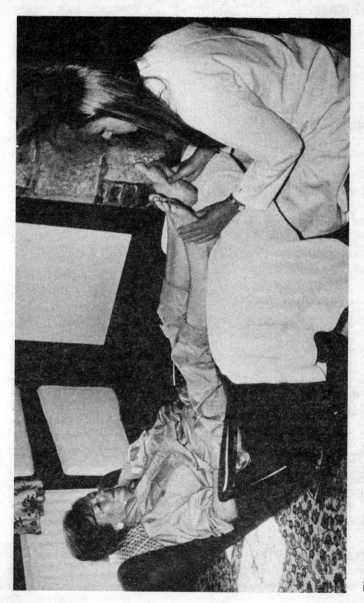

Figure 8.   The position for treatment.

after the removal of the patient's shoes and socks. This is the best position for a patient to be in, with the back comfortably supported and with the lower leg from knee to ankle also supported so that the feet can be rested in a relaxed and comfortable position. (See Figure 8.) If the knee is not bent and the leg is straight, the foot tends to be held more tensely which hampers the treatment. Another advantage of a recliner chair is that, although the body is well supported, the patient will be sitting at an angle which still allows the practitioner to see the face of the patient and note the various facial expressions and changes in colour. This is not possible if the patient lies flat on, for example, a massage couch. Another important factor for the practitioner is that the feet are supported high enough for him/her to work on them comfortably — just as with many occupations, a bad sitting position must be avoided to prevent back problems. When the patient is comfortably positioned, the treatment session will begin.

Examination of the Feet

To begin with, the practitioner will examine the feet. The general texture, temperature and colour of the feet will be noted first. Cold feet will indicate a poor circulation and feet which perspire a lot will indicate a glandular imbalance. If the skin is bluish or reddish in appearance, again a poor circulation may be indicated. The texture of the feet can also give an indication of the general condition of the body and if the skin of the feet is dry then this may indicate poor circulation and glandular imbalances.

Hard skin, corns, blisters, cracks, verrucas, athlete's foot, scars, puffiness and varicose veins will also be looked for. If such things as verrucas, athlete's foot or other infections are present then the area of the foot where they exist cannot be treated in case the infection is spread to other parts of the foot or picked up by the practitioner. If a large area of the foot is infected, the corresponding area on the hand can be treated instead. Areas of hard skin and corns may be the result of ill-fitting shoes, often the case with women keen to wear the various shoe fashions which may not always be beneficial to their feet! Posture can also affect the skin of the feet and areas of hard skin may indicate that the body's weight is not being evenly distributed through the feet, with additional weight on certain areas causing the thickening of the skin. Hard skin is also found on the feet of people who walk around bare-foot frequently and although this is good for the structure of the feet, the additional hard skin formed does make it difficult to contact the reflex areas in the feet. Varicosed areas would not be worked on since the veins might be further damaged by pressure, but scar tissue can be massaged gently and this may well have a beneficial effect on the area.

The condition of the tissues of the feet will also be examined. If there is swelling or puffiness of the foot, particularly around the ankles, this can relate to internal problems. If the feet are very tense, then this may indicate tension in the body and if the feet are rather limp with poor muscle tone, this may indicate a poor muscle tone throughout the body. Because of the presence of the zones in the feet and the fact that within the zones there is a flow of energy linking areas within the same zone, changes in the bone structure of the feet may relate to disturbances of the energy flow in the corresponding zone of the body. Hence, hammer toes (where the toes are joined at the lower joint) may indicate a problem in the head region or with the sinuses or teeth. An ingrowing toenail may relate to headaches or migraine and bunions (inflamed joints on the inner side of the foot) may indicate a cervical (neck) problem or even a thyroid problem. Flat feet, where the arch of the foot has dropped, may indicate a problem with the spine and if the cuneiform bones are sunken, there may be a problem with the small intestines.

With all of these problems in the feet, it is impossible to say whether the foot problem preceded the problem in the body or vice versa but a relationship can often exist. If the feet are in a poor condition the practitioner may well recommend the patient to visit a chiropodist for treatment, though sometimes problems with the feet themselves can be helped by reflexology treatment.

The Massage Technique

Before commencing to massage the feet, a small amount of talcum powder is applied to them as this allows easier movement from point to point. Oil is not used for this treatment as this would make the surface of the foot too slippery and sticky and, since the feet have a tendency to perspire, the talcum helps dry the feet slightly to ease treatment. Some practitioners prefer not to use talcum and this is quite acceptable. As the talcum is applied, the feet will be massaged in a general manner to help relax the patient.

The particular massage technique used for reflexology is different from other forms of massage and in the first instances of learning can be quite difficult to achieve. In general, the thumb is used to apply pressure to the various areas but the fingers may also be used. The thumb is held bent at a forty-five degree angle and the side and end of the thumb pressed firmly onto each reflex point — each reflex point is about the size of a pinhead so precision is required for the treatment to be effective (see Figure 9). While the thumb is pressed onto the reflex point, the other fingers will rest gently around the foot and the other hand will be used to support the area being worked on so will be resting on the opposite surface of the foot, i.e. when working with the thumb on points on the sole of the foot, the other hand will be resting on the top of the foot. After applying a firm pressure to the point being worked on, the pressure is then released by drawing the thumb back slightly but not losing contact with the foot. This slight drawing back then allows easier movement to the next reflex point to be worked on which will be reached by a half-circle movement forward to the next area. If pressure is to be applied to the same point, then after drawing the thumb back it is then pressed into the area again, thus using a circular movement on the point.

Both hands may be used and it is quite common for the practitioner to switch from using the right thumb to using the left thumb as it is easier to reach certain areas on each foot with one or other hand. Using this particular technique of keeping the thumb bent as much as possible prevents strain on the

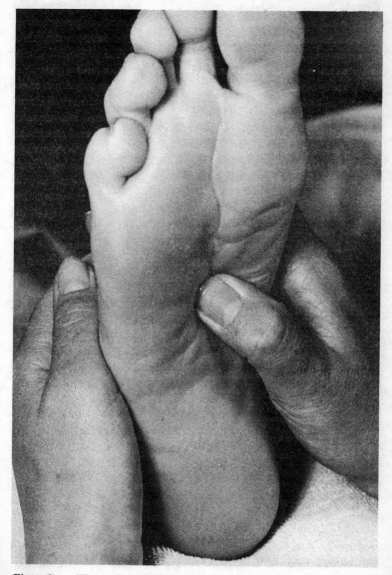

Figure 9. The angle of the thumb for applying the massage.

thumb joint and wrist which would result from a bending and
straightening of the thumb joint, though this method is
recommended by some authorities. The amount of pressure
applied to each point will vary from patient to patient and even
vary at different treatment sessions for the same patient
depending on their state of health. It is important that the
pressure applied is not agonizing to the patient as this would
immediately make him/her tense so the pressure will be firm
enough to feel like pressure which is bearable and is probably in
the region of 2 to 5 lb (1 to 2.3 kg).

Usually a pattern of treatment will be followed, commencing
with massage of the right foot with the reflexes to be found in
the region of the big toe. The whole foot will then be
systematically treated, working down from the toes across the
areas on the sole of the foot down to the heel. The areas on the
sides and top of the foot will then be treated before carrying out
the same procedure on the left foot. At the end of a complete
treatment both feet will be given some gentle manipulation and
the movements generally applied include rotation of the toes,
rotation of the ankles, a kneading action with the fist on the sole
of the foot and a wringing action with the hands cupped around
the sides of the foot and being rotated away from each other.
The treatment session will finish with a relaxing breathing
exercise where the thumbs are placed over the reflexes to the
solar plexus; as the patient breathes in pressure is applied to the
reflexes and the feet pushed up gently towards the body and as
the patient breathes out the pressure is released and the feet
pulled gently away from the body.

What the Treatment Feels Like
Some people say that they do not like their feet to be touched
and therefore could not possibly bear reflexology treatment! In
these cases, however, if the initial fear can be overcome, usually
the outcome is surprisingly pleasant! The other common fear is
that the treatment will tickle and it is not unusual for patients to
tell the practitioner that they are not sure that they will be able
to give them treatment since they are very ticklish! In nearly all

cases, however, the pressure applied is firm enough not to produce a ticklish sensation and occasionally when an area does appear to be ticklish, this often relates to a problem in the body area to which the underlying reflex area corresponds.

At different parts of the feet, different reactions are felt. Some areas when massaged may feel as if something very sharp, like a piece of glass or a thorn, is being pressed into the foot and patients often think that the practitioner is using his/her fingernail to apply the treatment, though this should not be the case with the conscientious practitioner who will have short fingernails to prevent this happening! In other areas the massage may produce a feeling of slight discomfort and in areas where definite crystals are present beneath the skin surface, the patient may be aware of these 'gritty' areas being worked on and slowly broken down. Around the ankle areas where the bones are more prominent, less pressure is required to contact the reflex points and if heavy pressure is used on these areas then the pain experienced may well be due to the actual pressure on the bones.

If there is much tension present in the body it is not surprising to find very many tender areas in the feet but those areas which are most tender will indicate which parts of the body are most out of balance. In some instances, on first receiving reflexology treatment, no tender areas are felt by the patient although he/she knows that there are areas in the body which are out of balance. This does not mean that the treatment is not going to be effective, provided that it has been applied correctly. With these instances it is often found that the feet become more sensitive with subsequent treatments as they become more responsive. This initial insensitivity usually occurs in people who are 'unaware' of their feet and it is almost as if an energy block has been formed to this area of the body which must be freed before the feet will respond to treatment. No response to the massage of the reflex areas may also be found sometimes in those with serious illnesses where there may be nerve damage or very poor circulation but, hopefully, these conditions will improve with treatment and the feet again become more responsive. In patients where there is paralysis of the lower leg and foot as may occur following a stroke and where no feeling is evident in the foot, it is interesting to find that sometimes these patients find the foot 'jerks' as the reflex areas are massaged, showing that nerve pathways are still intact.

Reactions from Treatment

Directly after a treatment session has finished the feet should feel warm and the patient should feel very relaxed. Since treatment is given first to one foot and then to the other foot, it is not uncommon for the practitioner to cover the completed foot with a towel to keep it warm while the other foot is being treated. Some people find the treatment so relaxing that they may actually fall asleep during the treatment session, particularly if they receive treatment at the end of a busy day. As the body can become so relaxed, it is best that the patient does not go dashing about directly after treatment to allow the relaxed state to continue and thus allow the healing processes in the body to take place more readily. Many patients do feel quite tired after a treatment and find it best to have a rest for about an hour afterwards. Other patients find that the treatment gives them a boost of energy and very often a feeling of wellbeing. Due to stimulation of the blood circulation, some patients feel very warm and sometimes flushed by the end of the session while the reverse effect can also occur, with the body directing the blood supply inwards to help with the healing processes and thus leaving the patient feeling cold and shivery for a short period after the treatment.

There will be no unpleasant side effects from reflexology — one reason why people are turning away from conventional medicine to the alternative therapies. It is possible, however, for some form of healing crisis to occur as the body attempts to heal itself and rid itself of toxic substances. The form of healing crisis which may occur will largely be determined by the imbalances which are present in the body and the degree of reaction will vary from person to person. Because of the possibility of a reaction to treatment occurring, the first treatment session will always be given quite gently to see how the person reacts — it is important not to cause too strong a reaction which may be distressing to the patient. It is better that the improvement be gained gradually with less stress on the body and it should be appreciated that, with most disorders, the effects have been building up over a period of time and an instantaneous improvement cannot be expected. The different forms of healing crisis will mainly affect the eliminating systems of the body which may show increased activity; these include the kidneys, the bowels, the skin and the lungs. The following are possible reactions which may occur following treatment:

(a)   there may be a more frequent desire to pass water as the kidneys react to secrete more urine, which may also vary in colour and odour.

(b)   there may be an increased activity of the bowels and possibly flatulence.

(c)   symptoms similar to those of a cold may appear as the mucous membranes of the nose, throat and lungs increase their secretions so the nose may need to be blown more often and coughing may increase with phlegm.

(d)   skin rashes may be aggravated especially in cases where rashes have been suppressed by medication and increased perspiration may occur.

(e)   in women, there may be an increased discharge from the vagina which may be more acid and cause a slight inflammation and irritation.

(f)   conditions of the past which have been suppressed may flare up.

(g)   sleep patterns may be disturbed with either deeper sleep or sometimes more difficulty with sleeping, and dreams may become more noticeable.

All of the listed reactions can be considered as positive factors, will be short-term and are indications that the body is attempting to become more balanced. Another reaction which has been known to occur following treatment is for the joints to become more flexible; in one particular case a lady always found that her fingers became 'double-jointed' after a treatment session!

Number of Treatments Required

The question of how many treatment sessions will be required by a patient for a condition to be righted is probably the most difficult to answer in relation to reflexology. Every patient is different and it is almost impossible to state in advance how many treatments will be necessary. It is often found that an immediate improvement occurs after the first session and this may be accounted for partly by a slight psychological factor of the patient enjoying the treatment and feeling that it is going to be of benefit. On the whole, results from treatment should become apparent after about three treatment sessions and these results may be of a complete improvement or of a considerable improvement of the condition. If there does not appear to be any difference noticeable to the patient after about three treatments, then it may be that reflexology is not going to be of help in this case. As a general guide, disorders which have been present for a long time will take longer to correct than those which have been present for a relatively short time and more serious disorders will also probably take a longer time to correct. For all conditions a course of treatment is required and even if just one session appears to have corrected the problem it is more sensible to have a short course of treatment to help balance up totally the body systems and to help prevent a recurrence of the disorder. For most conditions, a course of six to eight treatments is advisable and treatment sessions will usually take place at weekly intervals. Treatment may sometimes be given twice a week, particularly in conditions such as back problems, where considerable pain is being experienced. To treat more frequently than once or, on occasions twice, a week is not recommended since there is always the possibility of over-working an area and causing too strong a reaction in the body. It must be remembered that the body needs time to try to balance up the systems and for repair work to be done.

The length of time for each treatment session also varies but, since with every treatment all the reflex areas in both feet must be treated to treat the whole body, this will take about three-quarters of an hour. In certain cases where for reasons such as extremely sensitive feet or very tense feet it is then necessary to work more slowly, the treatment session may last up to one hour but to work for much longer than one hour is excessive. The advice of Eunice Ingham should always be remembered — that it is better to undertreat than overtreat. In a fairly healthy person where there are few tender reflex areas in the feet, less time may be required to give a complete treatment. It will be found that most reflexology practitioners allow one hour for each patient since this allows sufficient time to settle the patient comfortably, give the treatment and allow time for the patient to leave without feeling rushed.

When treating young children or babies, then obviously the length of time for the session will be less. In the first instance the feet are smaller so there is less area to be covered by the massage. Secondly, a child or baby is unlikely to sit quietly for an hour and would become restless near the end of a long treatment session, so an half-hour session will be sufficient. For children receiving treatment, it is usually a good idea if they are rather fidgety to allow them to bring something like a book or some pens and paper to keep their interest while the treatment is given, though some will sit quite peacefully for a complete session! Children do seem to enjoy the treatment and the results in these cases are often achieved quickly probably because the body has had less time to be thrown out of balance and is more responsive to righting itself. In one case known, a little boy so enjoyed his reflexology treatment and felt so much better afterwards that he would always insist on giving treatment himself to his mother when he got home!

Reflexology can thus be used as a means of treatment for men and women of all ages and is of benefit to nearly everyone to some degree, whether in completely correcting a disorder or in just making the person feel better in themselves and more relaxed. There are very few people who have experienced treatment properly administered and not benefited.

Chapter 4

The Reflex Areas

The way that the body can be divided into ten longitudinal and three transverse zone areas has already been described, as well as how these zones help to determine the position of the various reflex areas in the feet. Figure 10 shows the anatomical arrangement of the different parts of the body and the longitudinal zones in which these different parts are situated. The arrangement of the reflex areas in the feet will now be looked at more closely by considering the different systems of the body as follows:

1. The Head
2. The Musculo-Skeletal system
3. The Endocrine system
4. The Respiratory system
5. The Heart and Circulatory system
6. The Lymphatic system
7. The Digestive system
8. The Urinary system
9. The Skin

With each system, as well as describing where the corresponding reflex areas are found in the feet, there will also be a brief description of the functions of the different systems.

1. The Head
All the reflexes to the areas of the head are found in the regions of the toes, with the big toes also corresponding to all of the

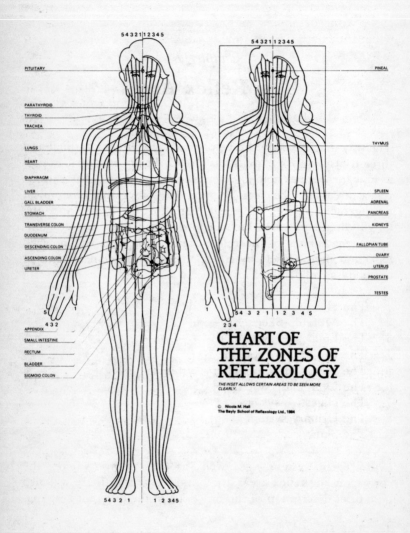

Figure 10.   The zone chart.

head and each big toe representing five zones.

The *brain* is part of the central nervous system of the body and is a most complex computer controlling a vast number of bodily functions. The brain is composed of a right and left hemisphere, with the right lobe controlling the left side of the body and the left lobe controlling the right side of the body. However, with reflexology the zone areas do not cross in the brain so that the right side of the brain is represented on the right foot and the left side of the brain is represented on the left foot. This is of particular importance when treating a condition such as a stroke where one side of the brain has experienced a haemorrhage, causing paralysis of the opposite side of the body — treatment will involve the reflex to the side of the brain in which the haemorrhage has occurred and the reflexes to the parts affected on the opposite side of the body and thus the opposite foot. From the brain there arise twelve cranial nerves which affect the sense of smell, taste, sight, hearing and motor functions involving the heart, lungs and abdominal organs so the brain area is of very great importance.

The reflex areas to the brain are found in the pads of the big toes, with the pituitary gland reflex approximately in the centre of the pad of the big toe and the top of the brain and top of the head reflex areas found at the top of the big toe just behind the nail. The reflex to the side of the brain and side of the head is found down the side of the big toe on the side nearest the second toe. The reflex to the face is found on the top surface of the big toe. (See Figure 11.)

The *sinuses* are hollow air-filled spaces in the cheekbones and behind the eyebrows and are linked with the nose. They are involved in giving resonance to the voice and also act as a protection to the eyes and the brain.

The reflexes to the sinuses are found in all four small toes on both feet not only all the way up the backs of these toes but sometimes also being more pronounced up the sides of the toes. Since the sinuses are found in zones two to five in the body, the reflexes are found in zones two to five in the feet. (See Figure 11.)

The *eyes* are the organs of vision and act in a similar manner to a camera with a lens focusing the light into the eye. This then passes to a light-sensitive screen at the back of the eye called the retina which can convert the light into an electrical impulse to be interpreted by the brain. The pupil of the eye, surrounded by the coloured iris, acts as an automatic light filter, the transparent window of the eye is self-cleansed by the tears and the eyelids act as a protective shutter.

The reflex to the eyes is found at the base of the second and third toes just below where these toes join the sole of the foot. The eyes in the body are situated in zones two and three so the reflexes in the feet are found in zones two and three, with the right eye represented in the right foot and the left eye represented in the left foot. (See Figure 11.)

The *ears* are the organs of hearing and, via the external and middle ear, sound vibrations can be interpreted as meaningful sounds. The bones of the middle ear, called the hammer, anvil and stirrup, are attached to the eardrum and are able to transmit vibrations to the inner ear. Within the inner ear an area called the cochlea translates the vibrations into nerve messages. Also within the inner ear are areas known as the semicircular canals which are responsible for maintaining balance.

The reflex to the ears is similarly placed to that of the reflex to the eyes but beneath the fourth and fifth toes, just below where these toes join the sole of the foot. The reflexes are thus in zones four and five, which are the zones in which the ears are positioned in the body. The right ear reflex is found on the right foot and the left ear reflex is found on the left foot. (See Figure 11.)

The *Eustachian tube* connects the middle ear to the back of the throat and is involved in keeping the air in the middle ear at atmospheric pressure. It is the tube that can become blocked when flying in an aeroplane and which can be unblocked by yawning or blowing the nose which helps equalize the pressures.

The reflex to the Eustachian tube is found between the eye and ear reflexes on the sole of the foot just below the web

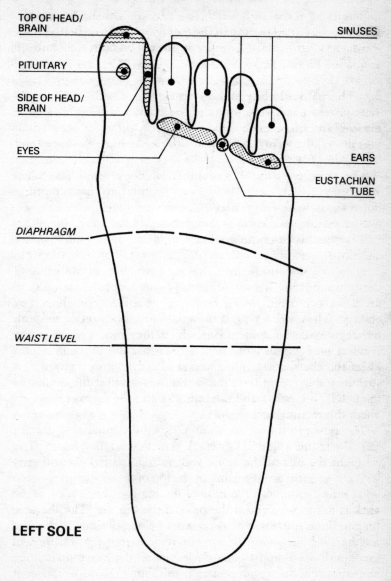

Figure 11.   The reflexes of the head on the sole of the left foot.

between the third and fourth toes. It can also be found in a similar position on the top of the foot below the web between the third and fourth toes. The reflex is present on both right and left feet. (See Figure 11.)

2. The Musculo-Skeletal System

This system covers the joints of the body and their associated muscles and includes the spine, the neck, the shoulder girdles, the elbows, the wrists, the pelvic girdles, the hips, the knees and the ankles.

The *spine* consists of a number of bony segments called vertebrae which can be divided into groups counting downwards, with seven cervical, twelve thoracic, five lumbar, five sacral and four coccygeal vertebrae. In the adult, the sacral and coccygeal vertebrae are fused to form two immobile bones called the sacrum and coccyx (the tailbone). The bony skeleton of the spine surrounds the spinal cord which is an extension of the brain and the nerves which originate from the spinal cord are named according to the region of the spine from which they emerge. These nerves affect the areas of the body on a level with the region of the spine from which they emerge. Thus the cervical nerves affect the neck and arms, the thoracic nerves affect the chest, the lumbar nerves affect the lower extremities such as the legs and feet, the sacral nerves affect the organs of the pelvis, the pelvis and the buttocks and the coccygeal nerves affect the rectum and anus.

The reflex to the spine is found down the inner side of both feet since the spine is situated centrally in the body. The different regions of the spine will be represented accordingly, with the cervical area starting at the top of the side of the big toe and ending level with the base of the big toe. The reflex to the neck is found all around the base of the big toe. The thoracic region of the spine will be represented along the side of the first metatarsal bone, with the lumbar region from the waistline of the foot down to approximately level with the inner ankle bone and the remaining area along the inner side of the foot representing the region of the sacrum and coccyx. (See Figure 12.)

RIGHT FOOT

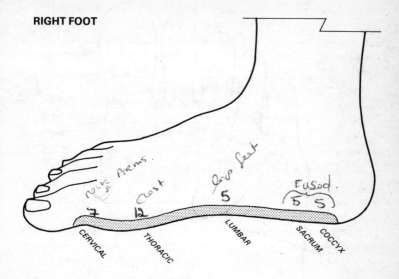

Figure 12. The reflexes of the spine on the side of the right foot.

The *upper limbs* have three main joints with the shoulders, the elbows and the wrists, in addition to the joints of the fingers.

The reflex to the shoulder is found around the base of the fifth (little) toe on the sole of the foot, the outer side of the foot and the top of the foot. The reflex area relating to the shoulder girdle will be found across the sole of the foot and the top of the foot in all five zones since the shoulder girdle exists in all five zones in the body. The reflex area will cover the upper half of the metatarsal bones and is in a similar area to that corresponding to the ribs, but in the latter case the reflex area will extend over the whole of the metatarsal bones. The reflex to the sternum (breastbone) is found on the top of the foot at the top end of the first metatarsal bone in zone one. (See Figure 13.)

The reflex to the upper arm can be found on the outer side of the foot, slightly on top of the foot leading down from the shoulder reflex to the base of the fifth metatarsal bone (the slight bony projection at waist level on the outer side of the foot), and

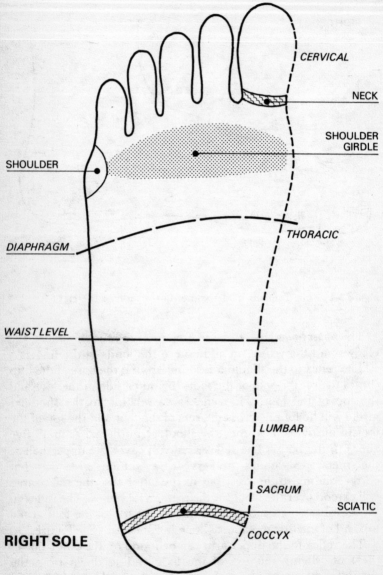

Figure 13. The reflexes of the musculo-skeletal system on the sole of the right foot and side of the left foot.

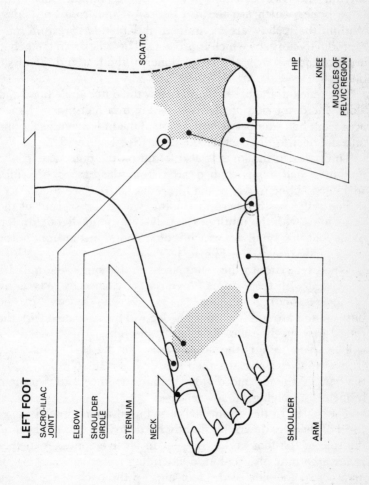

LEFT FOOT

SACRO-ILIAC JOINT

ELBOW

SHOULDER GIRDLE

STERNUM

NECK

SCIATIC

HIP

KNEE

MUSCLES OF PELVIC REGION

SHOULDER

ARM

the elbow reflex will be found actually the base of the fifth metatarsal bone. (See Figure 13.)

The *pelvis* is a large basin-shaped cavity formed by the sacrum and coccyx behind and by the innominate bones (the large bones which are the hip bones) at the front and sides. Within the pelvis are contained the bladder, rectum and reproductive organs which it protects. The reflexes to the pelvic areas are found over the tarsal bones of the feet and the ankle bones.

The reflex to the hip is found below the outer ankle bone and along the outer side of the foot mainly in a half-moon shaped area from half way between the base of the fifth metatarsal bone and the heel to the back of the heel. (See Figure 13.)

The reflex to the knee is also found on the outer side of the foot in a half-moon shaped area from the base of the fifth metatarsal bone to where the hip reflex starts. (See Figure 13.)

The reflex to the sacro-iliac joint (where the sacrum of the spine joins with the ilium of the pelvis) is found slightly on top of the foot in a small dip which is often found just in front of the outer ankle bone. (See Figure 13.)

When referring to the reflex areas to the joints, the muscles associated with these joints may also be reached by massaging the corresponding joint areas. Hence, the muscles of the buttock and around the top of the leg will be associated with the reflex areas to the sacro-iliac joints and hips.

The *sciatic nerve* is the largest nerve in the body and arises from the lower spine and then passes across the buttock, down the back of the leg and divides behind the knee into two main branches supplying the lower leg.

The reflex to the sciatic nerve is found approximately one-third of the way down the slightly hardened base of the heel on the sole of the foot and is present in all five zones. A further reflex area may also be found extending from the edges of this area across the side of the foot and up the back of the leg on either side of the Achilles tendon for a distance of a few inches.

Zone related area
In addition to the reflex areas of the feet, a development of the

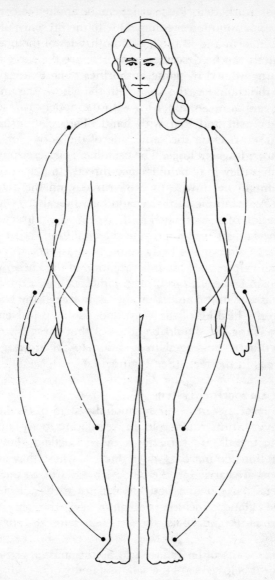

Figure 14. The zone-related areas.

4   REFLEXOLOGY

early 'hook work' described earlier can be applied in connection
with the upper and lower limbs. Due to the presence of the five
zones in the arm and in the leg on both sides of the body, zone
related areas can be described and these are the same as 'cross
reflexes' mentioned by some authorities. These areas link the
hip with the shoulder, the knee with the elbow, the ankle with
the wrist and also the upper leg with the upper arm, lower leg
with lower arm and foot with hand. The relationship exists
between the areas on the same side of the body, for instance
right elbow with right knee. The usefulness of these zone related
areas is that they may be massaged directly to help a condition
when it might be unwise to work directly on the actual area
affected. An example of this would be when there was severe
inflammation of a joint, such as the knee, when direct massage
to the knee might well aggravate the condition, but the elbow
on the same side of the body could be massaged directly and
might well help reduce the inflammation of the knee. A further
example can be applied to broken joints such as a broken wrist
where massage to the ankle, on the same side of the body, may
speed up the healing of the wrist and also help prevent severe
muscle wasting. It should be stressed that these zone related
areas would be massaged in addition to the massage of the
reflex areas in the feet. (See Figure 14.)

3.   The Endocrine System
The endocrine system is the hormonal system of the body and
plays a very important role in regulating body functions.
Endocrine glands are sometimes called ductless glands since
their secretions do not pass down ducts to where they are to act
but instead are carried in the blood-stream around the body to
the various parts of the body which are to be affected. The
endocrine glands include the pituitary, the thyroid, the
parathyroids, the adrenals, the pancreas and the reproductive
glands.

The *pituitary* is often referred to as the master gland of the
body since it helps control the action of many of the other glands
in the body. Although only a tiny gland, about the size of a pea,

it can be divided anatomically into an anterior and posterior part, with each part producing a number of different hormones. The hormones produced by the pituitary affect growth (an imbalance can result in gigantism or dwarfism), affect the secretions of the thyroid, adrenals and reproductive glands (thus affecting metabolism, blood pressure, water balance, sexual development and reproduction) and affect the muscles of the uterus and mammary glands in the pregnant woman. The pituitary hormones also have many other functions.

The reflex to the pituitary gland is found in the centre of the pad of the big toe though it may vary slightly in position being somewhat higher or lower or more to one side. This reflex is found to be tender in most people and this can probably be explained by the fact that the pituitary gland is involved in so many functions as the master gland and that the hormonal system which it controls is so easily thrown out of balance by tension and stress which are present in a great many people. Although there is only one pituitary gland in the body, a reflex to the pituitary will be found in both big toes. (See Figure 15.)

The *thyroid* is a two-lobed gland situated in the neck with a thin area called the isthmus joining the two lobes to give this gland the shape of a bow-tie. The main role of the thyroid gland is to control the metabolic rate in the body (the rate at which cell activity takes place with the production of heat and energy). By the production of the hormone thyroxine from the gland, the rate of cell metabolism can be increased. When the gland is overactive or underactive, various physical and mental changes can occur. Another hormone produced by the thyroid is calcitonin, which affects the blood calcium levels and works in opposition to the hormone produced by the parathyroid glands. Calcitonin acts to increase the calcium uptake by the bones.

The reflex to the thyroid gland is found in both feet in zone one since the gland is situated in zone one in the neck. The right lobe will be represented in the right foot and the left lobe will be represented in the left foot. The thyroid area is over the ball of the big toe and more particularly in the upper part of this area. (See Figure 15.)

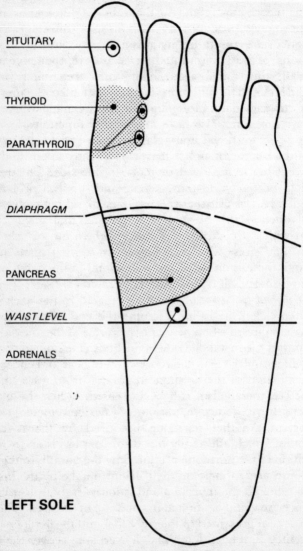

PITUITARY

THYROID

PARATHYROID

DIAPHRAGM

PANCREAS

WAIST LEVEL

ADRENALS

LEFT SOLE

Figure 15. The reflexes of the endocrine system on the sole of the left foot.

The *parathyroids* are two pairs of small glands embedded in the back of the thyroid gland in the neck. Although situated so closely to the thyroid, their function is separate and these glands produce a hormone called parathyroid hormone which acts to control the levels of calcium and phosphorus in the blood.

The reflexes to the parathyroid glands are found associated with the reflex to the thyroid gland in both feet in the area of the ball of the big toe but on the border of zone one and zone two, i.e. on a level with a line drawn straight down on the sole of the foot from the web between the big toe and second toe. An upper and lower parathyroid reflex will be found in both feet corresponding to the upper and lower glands on both sides of the body. (See Figure 15.)

The *adrenals* are situated on top of each kidney in the body, rather more to the medial side. Each adrenal gland can be divided into an outer area called the cortex and an inner area called the medulla. The adrenal medulla produces the hormones adrenalin and noradrenalin. Adrenalin is the hormone associated with 'fear, flight and fight' since its role is to prepare the body for action in these conditions. The effect of adrenalin is to increase the blood supply to the areas in need, such as the brain, the muscles, the heart and the lungs and to decrease the blood supply to areas such as the skin and digestive tract which are not so vital at these times. It also increases the heart rate and blood pressure and causes the release of glucose to supply extra energy. The adrenal cortex produces hormones which influence carbohydrate metabolism and the mineral balance in the body and it also produces additional sex hormones. Through the various hormones which it produces, the adrenal gland can also influence the muscle tone of the body, help reduce inflammation, aid against allergic reactions and help the body cope with stress and fatigue. Since the adrenal hormones are probably involved in over fifty different functions, the adrenal gland is of great importance.

The reflexes to the adrenal glands are found just above and slightly to the inner side of the kidney reflexes in zone two of the feet, a little above the waist level of the soles of the feet. The right adrenal gland will be represented in the right foot and the left adrenal gland will be represented in the left foot. (See Figure 15.)

The *pancreas* is unique in that it is both an endocrine gland and an exocrine gland. The exocrine function is the production of digestive juices which pass down the pancreatic duct into the small intestine and this function will be discussed under the digestive system on p.72. The endocrine function is the production of insulin which acts to lower the blood sugar level. It is important for the blood sugar level to be precisely regulated since glucose is the main energy source which can be utilized by the brain. The region of the pancreas called the Islets of Langerhans which produces insulin can also produce another substance called glucagon which can produce an increase in the blood sugar level, so both the hormones produced are involved in carbohydrate metabolism. In the body the pancreas is situated behind the stomach just above the waistline.

The reflex to the pancreas is found in both the right and left feet just above the waistline and below the diaphragm in zones one and two on the right foot and zones one, two and three on the left foot. Since in the body the stomach overlaps the pancreas, in the feet the stomach reflex overlaps the reflex to the pancreas on the soles of the feet. (See Figure 15.)

The *reproductive glands* of the female are the ovaries and of the male are the testes. The ovaries produce the hormones oestrogen and progesterone which are responsible for the development at puberty of the secondary sex characteristics. After puberty in the female a cyclical production of ova (the female germ cells) continues until the menopause, unless pregnancy or disease occurs. The ovarian hormones produce regular changes in the fallopian tubes, uterus and vagina throughout the menstrual cycle. The testes produce spermatozoa (the male germ cells) and the hormone testosterone which, with the androgens produced by the adrenal cortex, is responsible for the development at puberty of the secondary sex organs and secondary sex characteristics. The two ovaries are situated on either side in the pelvis and are

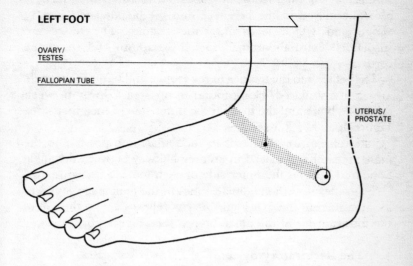

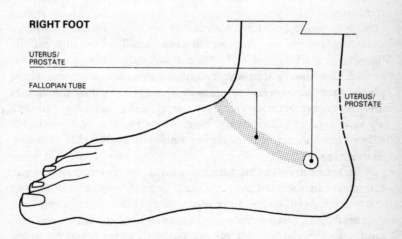

Figure 16.   The reflexes of the reproductive system on the sides of the feet.

connected via the fallopian tubes to the uterus, which is centrally placed in the pelvis behind the bladder and slightly above and which leads into the vagina. The testes are suspended extra-abdominally by the scrotum and spermatic cords.

The reflexes to the ovaries in the female and testes in the male are similarly placed, being found in an area halfway between the ankle bone and the heel on the outer side of each foot. (See Figure 16.)

The reflexes to the uterus in the female and prostate in the male are similarly placed in an area halfway between the ankle bone and heel on the inner side of each foot. (See Figure 16.)

The reflexes to the fallopian tubes in the female are found in an area linking the ovary and uterus reflexes across the top of the foot in front of the ankle bones. (See Figure 16.)

4.   The Respiratory System

The respiratory system comprises the nose and mouth, the throat, the larynx, the trachea (the windpipe), the bronchi and the lungs.

The *lungs* are tree-like in structure with two main branches, the bronchi, dividing into smaller and smaller branches called bronchioles before ending in the air sacs called the alveoli. It is within the alveoli that the essential exchange of gases takes place, with the oxygen breathed in being taken up by the blood and the carbon dioxide from the blood being taken up into the air sacs to be breathed out. There are two lungs, one on either side of the thoracic cavity, being enclosed by the ribs and the diaphragm.

The reflex areas to the lungs are found in both feet across all five zones in the area over the metatarsal bones, and both the soles and tops of the feet may show reflex areas. (See Figure 17.)

The *bronchi, trachea, larynx, throat, nose* and *mouth* are all air conducting passages and no exchange of gases takes place in these areas.

The reflexes to the bronchi and the trachea are found leading down from the web between the big toe and second toe into the lung area and are present on both the sole and top of the right and left feet. (See Figure 17.)

The reflexes to the nose and throat will be found on the top of the big toe in an area just above where the toe joins the foot. (See Figure 17.)

The *diaphragm* is a dome-shaped sheet of muscle which separates the thorax from the abdomen and encloses the lower surface of the lungs. The mechanism of breathing is a muscular action which involves the movement of the diaphragm. During inspiration the diaphragm contracts and descends, increasing the capacity of the thorax, while during expiration the diaphragm relaxes and ascends, decreasing the capacity of the thorax.

The reflex area to the diaphragm is found on both feet on the soles, following a line across at the lower level of the ball of the big toe and across the ball of the foot. (See Figure 17.)

The *solar plexus* is a network of nerves giving off branches to all parts of the abdominal cavity; it is situated just in front of the diaphragm and behind the stomach. It is sometimes called the 'abdominal brain' since it supplies the abdominal areas as well as the diaphragm and adrenal glands. It is thus a useful area for the relief of tension, stress, fright, anger and nervousness.

The reflex to the solar plexus will be found in a similar area to that of the diaphragm on the soles of the feet, but particularly in zones two and three on both feet. (See Figure 17.)

5.   The Heart and Circulatory System

A healthy circulation is vital for the good health of all parts of the body and when working on the reflex areas in the feet, the circulation to the corresponding part of the body will be improved.

The *heart* is a muscular pump which sends the blood around the circulatory system through a series of vessles called arteries, capillaries and veins. The arteries carry oxygenated blood to the tissues where an exchange of materials takes place in the capillary beds and the deoxygenated blood is then returned to the heart via the veins. This blood is then circulated to the lungs

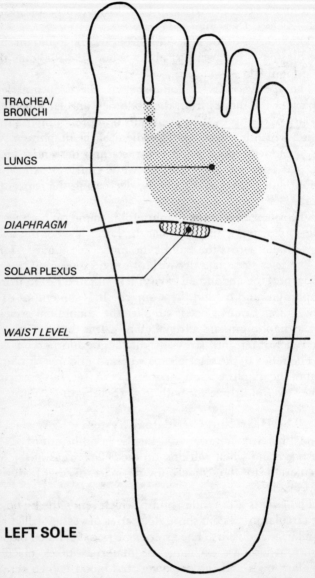

TRACHEA/
BRONCHI

LUNGS

DIAPHRAGM

SOLAR PLEXUS

WAIST LEVEL

LEFT SOLE

Figure 17. The reflexes of the respiratory system on the sole and top of the left foot.

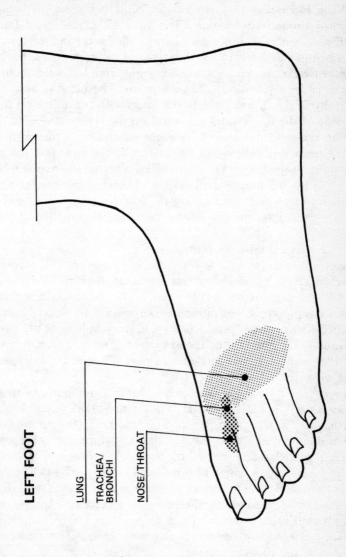

LEFT FOOT

LUNG

TRACHEA/
BRONCHI

NOSE/THROAT

where carbon dioxide is given up and more oxygen collected and the blood then returns to the heart before again being pumped around the system. The heart is made up of four chambers, with the upper ones being called atria and the lower ones being called ventricles. A system of valves prevents back-flow between the chambers with right and left sides being separated by a partition called a septum. The heart is situated centrally in the thorax close to the lungs with two-thirds on the left side of the thorax and one-third on the right side.

The reflex to the heart is a slight exception to the normal determination of reflex areas according to the zone position of the organ in the body. The main reflex area to the heart will be found in the left foot in zones two and three above the level of the diaphragm and overlapping the lower area relating to the left lung reflex on the sole of the foot. (See Figure 18.)

6. The Lymphatic System

The lymphatic system is also a circulatory system which works closely with the blood system but is separate from it. Lymphatic vessels are present throughout the body and contain a fluid called lymph which is similar in composition to blood plasma and contains waste products of cell metabolism which are eventually returned to the blood system. The main function of the lymphatic system is its role as part of the body's defence mechanism.

Lymph nodes are aggregates of lymphatic tissue found in areas along the lymphatic vessels. The lymph nodes are found particularly in the groin, the armpit, the neck, the breast and the abdomen and within these nodes the lymph is filtered and foreign particles and infectious material is ingested by cells called lymphocytes which thus helps to purify the lymph before it is returned to the blood system via the right and left subclavian veins found in the neck. In certain conditions, the lymph nodes can become enlarged.

The reflexes to the upper lymph nodes are found on the top of the feet at the roots of the toes. (See Figure 19.)

The reflexes to the lymph nodes of the breast are found on the

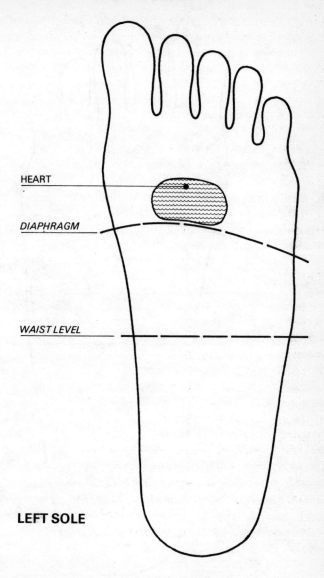

Figure 18. The reflex of the heart.

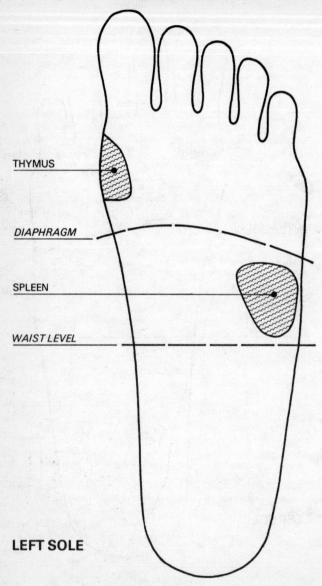

THYMUS

DIAPHRAGM

SPLEEN

WAIST LEVEL

LEFT SOLE

Figure 19.   The reflexes of the lymphatic system on the sole and
top of the left foot.

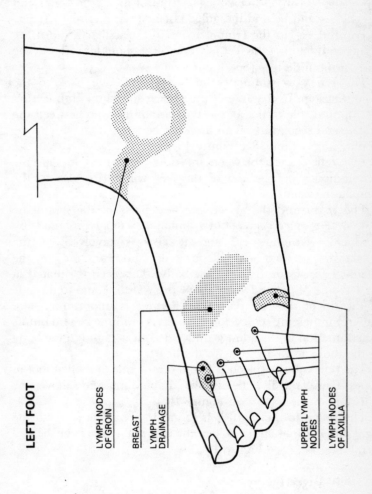

LEFT FOOT

LYMPH NODES OF GROIN

BREAST

LYMPH DRAINAGE

UPPER LYMPH NODES

LYMPH NODES OF AXILLA

top of the feet in zones two, three and four in the thoracic region lying over the metatarsal bones. (See Figure 19.)

The reflexes to the lymph nodes of the groin are found on the top of the feet in all five zones in front of the ankle bones and also below and behind the ankle bones. (See Figure 19.)

The reflexes to the lymph nodes of the axilla (armpit) are found on the top of the feet just below the shoulder reflex at the base of the little toe. (See Figure 19.)

The reflex to stimulate the lymph drainage back to the venous system in the area of the neck is found on both feet on the top and sole of the foot at the base of the web between the big toe and second toe. This area can be worked on with a type of pinching action. (See Figure 19.)

The reflex areas between the areas described for specific lymph nodes on the top of the feet will relate also to the lymphatic system.

The *spleen* and the *thymus* are also parts of the lymphatic system. The spleen can act in a similar way to a lymph node by producing lymphocytes, and it also is involved in the breakdown of old red blood cells and can recycle the haemoglobin from these. In the body, the spleen is situated in the left side of the abdomen above the waistline and to the side of the tip of the pancreas. The thymus is important before puberty in helping to develop the body's immune system but its exact function in the adult is undecided. It is found in the body in the thoracic cavity close to the heart.

The reflex to the spleen is found on the sole of the left foot in zones four and five below the diaphragm and above the waistline of the foot. (See Figure 19.)

The reflex to the thymus is found in zone one on both the right and left foot on the sole of the foot in an area over the ball of the big toe. (See Figure 19.)

7.   The Digestive System

The digestive system is responsible for breaking down the molecules of food ingested into particles that can be absorbed by the blood and which can then be used for the various bodily processes. Any undigested food passes through the digestive system and is expelled. The food ingested passes into the mouth, then down the oesophagus to the stomach, and then to the small intestine and large intestine, with the residue being expelled through the rectum and anus. The liver, gall bladder and pancreas are also involved with the process of digestion.

The *oesophagus* leads from the mouth to the stomach and is a muscular tube acting as a passageway to the more important areas where digestion will be carried out.

The reflex to the oesophagus is found on the sole of the foot leading down from the web between the big toe and second toe along the area over the sides of the first and second metatarsal bones to the stomach area. This reflex may also be found on the top of the foot. (See Figure 20.)

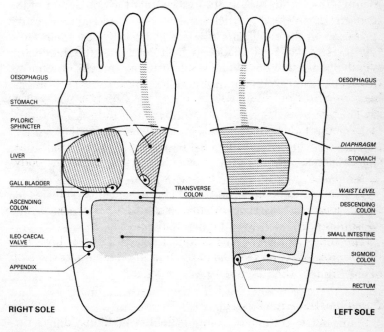

Figure 20. The reflexes of the digestive system on the sole of the right and left foot.

The *stomach* is a sac-like structure found in the upper abdomen above waist level on both right and left sides of the body, but with the major part of the stomach more to the left. In this area, food is mixed with digestive juices but no main absorption takes place.

The reflex to the stomach is found on both left and right feet on the soles of the feet above the waistline of the foot and below the diaphragm level. It is found mainly in zones one, two and three in the left foot and zone one on the right foot. (See Figure 20.)

The *small intestine* receives food from the stomach and the two are separated by the pyloric sphincter which controls the flow of food between them. The small intestine can be divided into three main parts called the duodenum, the jejunum and the ileum. It is within the small intestine that the absorption of the broken down food particles takes place and the digestive processes of the small intestine are assisted by secretions from the pancreas and gall bladder which enter into the duodenum via the pancreatic duct. The small intestine consists of some six to seven metres of tubing doubled back on itself in the abdomen.

The reflex to the small intestine is found in both feet on the sole of the foot below the waistline of the foot and extending down in the area over the tarsal bones in zones one, two, three and four. (See Figure 20.)

The *large intestine* commences with an area called the caecum and an important valve called the ileo-caecal valve regulates the passage of food from the ileum of the small intestine to the caecum. The large intestine then passes up the right side of the body with the ascending colon which bends round beneath the liver at approximately waist level to become the transverse colon which continues across to the left side of the abdomen to below the spleen where it becomes the descending colon. This area continues down the left side before turning towards the midline and becoming the sigmoid colon which then leads to the rectum. The rectum is centrally positioned and leads into the anus. The bend in the large intestine below the liver is referred to as the hepatic flexure and the bend below the spleen is referred to as the splenic flexure. The appendix is situated off the lower end of the caecum. The main function of the large intestine is to absorb water and salts to conserve the body fluids and it also stores the waste faecal matter until it is expelled.

The reflexes to the regions of the large intestine are found on the soles of both the right and left foot. Commencing on the right foot in zones four and five in the area over the lower tarsal bones with the appendix and ileo-caecal valve reflexes, the ascending colon reflex is found leading up from this area to the waistline of the foot. The transverse colon reflex is found in all ten zones at waist level, with the descending colon reflex found in the left foot similarly placed to the ascending colon reflex in the right foot. The reflex to the sigmoid colon follows an S-shaped path from the end of the descending colon reflex to the inner side of the left foot where the reflex to the rectum is found. A reflex to the rectum may also be found extending from this area up the back of the leg for a short distance on either side of the Achilles tendon. (See Figure 20.)

The *liver* is the largest gland in the body and amongst its functions are the processes of detoxification, storage of carbohydrates, proteins, fats, vitamins and minerals and the production of bile. In the body, the liver extends across all five zones on the right side and zones one, two and three on the left side between the diaphragm and the waist.

The reflex to the liver is found predominantly in the right foot in zones three, four and five of the sole of the foot between the level of the diaphragm and the waist. The reflex is not so evident in the other zones which relate to the position of the liver in the body. (See Figure 20.)

The *gall bladder* is attached to the lower right lobe of the liver and stores the bile produced by the liver. The bile will be released down the bile duct into the duodenum of the small intestine to assist in the absorption of dietary fat and fat-soluble vitamins.

The reflex to the gall bladder is found in the right foot in zone three just below the liver reflex and thus just above the waist level of the sole of the foot. (See Figure 20.)

The *pancreas*, as described in the previous section on the endocrine system, produces various digestive enzymes which pass along the pancreatic duct which joins with the bile duct to enter into the duodenum of the small intestine. The enzymes act on the proteins, carbohydrates and fats to break them down into smaller molecules which can be more readily absorbed from the small intestine. The pancreas lies across the posterior abdominal wall behind the stomach, with the head of the pancreas situated in the concavity of the C-shaped duodenum.

The reflex to the pancreas is found below the diaphragm level and above the waist level in zones one and two on the sole of the right foot and zones one, two and three on the sole of the left foot. (See Figure 15.)

8. The Urinary System

The urinary system is made up of a right and left kidney each connected by a ureter tube to the bladder. This is the main excretory system of the body.

The *kidneys* act as a filtering system which works to maintain the composition and volume of the body fluids. Each kidney is made up of approximately one million microscopic units, called nephrons, which are responsible for the formation of urine. The kidneys are positioned on the posterior abdominal wall at about waist level in zones two and three. The left kidney is situated slightly higher than the right kidney.

The reflexes to the kidneys are found in the soles of the feet at about waist level in zones two and three with the right kidney reflex in the right foot and the left kidney reflex in the left foot. (See Figure 21.)

The *ureter tubes* are long, thin muscular tubes which convey urine from the kidneys to the bladder.

The reflexes to the ureter tubes are found in the soles of the feet joining the kidney reflex to the bladder reflex and thus passing from zones three and two across and down to zone one at the inner side of the feet. (See Figure 21.)

The *bladder* is a hollow muscular organ which acts as a

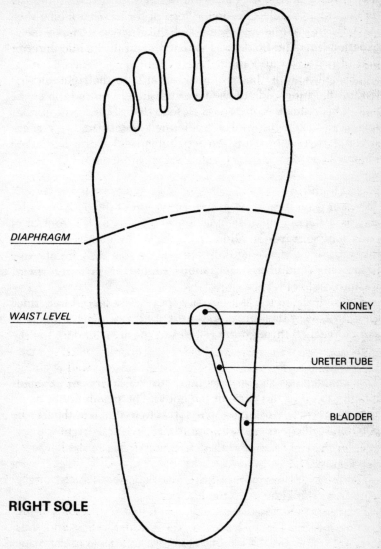

DIAPHRAGM

WAIST LEVEL

KIDNEY

URETER TUBE

BLADDER

RIGHT SOLE

Figure 21. The reflexes of the urinary system on the sole of the right foot.

reservoir for the urine. The urine which is formed continuously by the kidneys collects drop by drop in the bladder which then expands in volume and when full the desire to pass urine is experienced. The bladder is situated centrally in the anterior part of the lower abdomen.

The reflex to the bladder is found in both the right and left foot on the inner side of the foot and slightly on the top of the foot. This reflex in zone one is close to that of the lower lumbar region of the spine and is sometimes identified by a slight swelling in this area on the top inner side of the foot. (See Figure 21.)

9.   The Skin

The skin is an important excretory system of the body and also acts as a barrier against infection and helps in the control of body temperature. In addition to the many glands present in the skin, many nerve endings are also present allowing the five basic skin (cutaneous) sensations of touch, pressure, pain, warmth and cold.

The reflexes to the skin are not specifically placed but, since the skin covers the entire body, the different areas of the skin can be reached through the reflexes to the areas underlying the skin.

This chapter has shown how there are reflex areas in the feet relating to all of the parts of the body. The possibility of being able to treat all of these parts through the feet offers the potential to help very many disorders.

Chapter 5

What Reflexology is Most Effective in Treating

By being able to treat all the different parts of the body through the feet, due to the fact that reflex areas to all these different parts exist in the feet, reflexology does offer itself as a potential treatment for nearly all disorders. Often people deciding to try a form of alternative medicine find it difficult to decide which method would be best, since nearly all the alternative therapies treat the body as a whole and offer an opportunity of helping most disorders. The choice must, therefore, lie with the patient who must decide which treatment they fancy and this decision may well be affected by the availability of the different practitioners in their area. In addition, some people may be put off by the idea of having needles inserted into their skin as in acupuncture, and some people may prefer the idea of actually taking some form of medication as with homoeopathy, herbalism and vitamin therapy since they are more accustomed to the idea of taking something to make them feel better. Others may not like the idea of having their feet touched! Once a particular type of therapy has been selected then a course of this treatment will be required and regular treatment sessions will be essential. It is not sensible to imagine that in any therapy a 'one-off' treatment is going to correct problems which may have been present or may have been developing over several years and any treatment must be given a fair try to see if it will be effective.

To help understand the type of conditions which may be treated by reflexology treatment, some of the more common conditions seen by practitioners will now be discussed. It is important to remember that with reflexology, whatever the condition being treated, all the different reflex areas in the feet will be massaged. However, in certain conditions, certain reflex areas are obviously going to be of greater importance in helping to balance up the body and these areas will thus require extra massage. In general, when giving reflexology treatment, any reflex area which the patient finds tender when massaged will be given extra massage. When the full treatment has been given, the practitioner will return to the areas which showed tenderness. After further massage they will appear in many cases to be less tender than when initially worked on. By being able to treat the whole body through the feet, not only can symptoms be helped but also the cause of the symptoms.

With each condition to be discussed under the various systems of the body the direct reflex areas involved (DR) and their associated reflex areas (AR) will be mentioned. The direct reflex areas will relate to the main symptoms experienced in a condition and the main body area or areas involved in that condition. The associated reflex areas will relate to areas which can be, though are not necessarily, involved in the condition and may also relate to its cause.

1. The Head

Headaches and Migraine: these may be caused by a number of different factors including tension, neck problems, sinus congestion, eye trouble, food or other allergies, poor diet and in women may be associated with the hormonal changes which take place during the menstrual cycle and the menopause.

DR : head , big toe areas.

AR : neck, cervical spine, sinuses, eyes, solar plexus, stomach, small and large intestine, liver, gall bladder, reproductive glands.

Stroke (Cerebral haemorrhage): a haemorrhage (clot) on one side of the cerebral area of the brain can cause total or partial paralysis of the opposite side of the body.

DR : head, big toe areas, spine, areas affected such as arm, leg.

AR : heart, solar plexus, adrenal glands.

Parkinson's disease: this disorder affects the fore-brain and causes an involuntary movement of the muscles leading to the characteristic tremor of the hands and shuffled walk which occurs.
DR : head, big toe areas.
AR : spine, adrenal glands, large intestine.

Multiple sclerosis: a deterioration of the protective covering of the nerves in the brain and spinal cord which can lead to visual and speech disturbances, loss of balance and co-ordination, muscle weakness with paralysis and bladder and bowel disturbances.
DR : head, big toe areas, spine.
AR : adrenal glands, large intestine, bladder, eyes.

Sinusitis and Catarrh: congestion in the sinus region due to an excess of mucus. If there is infection or inflammation present the condition is known as sinusitis. The congestion may also lead to headaches.
DR : sinuses, big toe areas, eyes.
AR : ileo-caecal valve, adrenal glands, upper lymphatics.

Hay fever: inflammation of the nasal mucus membranes due to an allergy to pollen. As well as the nose, the eyes and throat can also be affected and treatment for this condition is best given for a period before the time of year when the person is affected, this may help prevent the symptoms occurring or lessen the symptoms.
DR : sinuses, big toe areas, eyes.
AR : ileo-caecal valve, adrenal glands, lungs (bronchi), spleen, upper lymphatics.

Eye disorders: a general improvement of the eyesight often occurs with reflexology treatment. Other conditions such as *blocked tear ducts* (dry eyes), *watery eyes, cataracts* (loss of transparency of lens of eye), *conjunctivitis* (inflammation of the conjunctiva covering the eyeball) and *glaucoma* (increase in pressure of fluid in front of the lens of the eye leading to hardening of the eyeball) may also be helped. With the more serious conditions, the results will be better if the conditions are treated in the early stages of their development.

DR : eyes.
AR : neck, cervical spine, kidneys, adrenal glands, upper
	lymphatics.

Ear disorders: hearing problems due to nerve damage or catarrh
may often be helped, but deafness due to structural damage to
the ear or where surgery has been carried out may not be so
successfully treated. *Tinnitus* is a condition where noises of
varying intensities are experienced in the ear. The exact cause
of this condition is not known but it may be associated with
catarrhal congestion, tension in the head area or inflammation
or infection of the delicate ear mechanism. Whatever the cause,
this is an extremely stressful condition. *Ménière's disease* involves
the inner ear and can cause deafness, noises in the ear, loss of
balance and giddiness and nausea.
DR : ears.
AR : neck, cervical spine, big toes areas (particularly side of
	big toe next to second toe), sinuses and Eustachian tube
	(for catarrhal deafness), solar plexus, adrenal glands,
	upper lymphatics.

Toothache: this can sometimes be temporarily relieved using the
reflex areas to the teeth.

2.   The Musculo-Skeletal System
Spinal (back) problems: the treatment will not be able to diagnose
the exact nature of the back problem but help can be given in
many cases, including a *slipped disc, pulled muscle, curvature of the
spine* and *stiffness in the back.*
DR : spine (region affected).
AR : adrenal glands, areas supplied by nerves from region of
	spine affected, solar plexus.

Neck problems
DR : neck, cervical spine.
AR : rotation of big toe to help ease neck, solar plexus, adrenal
	glands.

Shoulder problems: these may include a *frozen shoulder, stiffness, pins*

and needles from the shoulder down the arm. Problem involving the shoulder are often associated with problems with the neck.
DR : shoulder, shoulder girdle.
AR : neck, cervical spine, rotation of big toe, arm, solar plexus.

Tennis elbow and Golfer's elbow: the pain in these two similar conditions affects opposite sides of the elbow joint.
DR : elbow.
AR : shoulder, arm, neck, cervical spine, knee and massage to knee directly (as zone related area), adrenal glands.

Lower back problems
DR : lumbar and sacral spine, coccyx.
AR : sacro-iliac joint, hip, muscles of pelvic region, sciatic regions, adrenal glands, solar plexus.

Hip problems
DR : hip.
AR : lower spine, sacro-iliac joint, muscles of pelvic region, sciatic regions, adrenal glands, solar plexus.

Sciatica: in this condition pain is experienced along the path of the sciatic nerve either along the whole area of the nerve or just a part of the area. The nerve can be affected by inflammation, pressure on the nerve at the level of the spine where it originates or pressure on the nerve due to the pelvis being out of alignment, poor posture such as may be caused by arthritis in a hip, swelling of an abdominal organ, pregnancy or obesity.
DR : sciatic regions.
AR : lower spine, sacro-iliac joint, hip, muscles of pelvic region, abdominal organs, solar plexus.

Arthritis and Rheumatism: arthritis is a condition which causes pain and inflammation of the joints, while rheumatism refers to a group of conditions where there may be pain, stiffness and swelling of muscles and joints. Both terms cover a number of more specific disorders. It is usually found that these conditions tend to affect the body in general as well as specific areas, so a good general treatment is required.

DR : joints and muscles directly affected, direct massage to zone related areas.

AR : pituitary, parathyroid glands, kidneys, solar plexus.

Gout: this is a form of arthritis mostly affecting the big toe joint, which becomes shiny, swollen, red and extremely sore. The wrists, ankles and thumbs can also be affected. In this condition an excess of uric acid is found in the blood.

DR : joint affected through zone related area.

AR : solar plexus, kidneys, adrenal glands.

3. The Endrocrine System

Pituitary disorders: apart from conditions where the pituitary gland is directly affected by, for instance, a tumour, the reflex to this gland will be important when treating a condition involving the other endocrine glands. The reflex will also be helpful when treating fevers, fainting and some kidney disorders.

Thyroid disorders: with an *over-active thyroid* gland, the symptoms may include restlessness, nervousness, irritability, tiredness, weight loss but with an appetite and, in more pronounced cases, there may be protrusion of the eyes. With an *under-active thyroid* gland, there is a general slowing down of the metabolic processes with possible symptoms of weight gain, sluggishness, shortness of breath, weakness and tiredness. A *goitre* is a swelling of the thyroid gland.

DR : thyroid.

AR : pituitary, reproductive glands.

Parathyroid gland disorders: since the hormone produced by this gland is involved in the regulation of the blood calcium level, the reflexes will be important in conditions where this level is at fault with a resultant effect on nerve and muscle functions. It will be important in helping problems with *cramps* and also *arthritis* and cases of *kidney and gall stones.*

Adrenal gland disorders: due to the many functions of the adrenal hormones produced, the reflexes to the adrenal glands will be important in conditions involving the adrenal hormones, such as disorders of the metabolism of fats, proteins and carbohydrates, disorders of the salt and water balance in the body, kidney problems, blood pressure disorders, sex hormone problems and conditions of stress, inflammation, muscle tone and allergies.

Pancreas disorders: the main disorder involving the pancreas is *diabetes*, where an increased blood sugar level occurs due to insufficient insulin. In addition to the disturbance in carbohydrate metabolism, structural changes may also develop in the kidneys, eyes, blood vessels and nerves with diabetes. *Hypoglycaemia* occurs in the reverse situation when the blood sugar level becomes too low.
DR : pancreas.
AR : adrenal glands, pituitary gland, kidneys, liver, eyes.

Particular care is required with the treatment of diabetes with reflexology due to the possible effect of the alteration of the amount of insulin produced by the pancreas.

Reproductive gland disorders:
(a) *Female problems:* many women suffer with *problems concerned with the menstrual cycle, infertility* and the *menopause.* Premenstrual tension, pain at the time of ovulation, irregular periods and other symptoms can all often be helped. Extra care is required in treating problems of the female reproductive glands and it is not uncommon for irregularities of the menstrual cycle to occur as a result of treatment as the body becomes balanced.
DR : ovaries, Fallopian tubes, uterus.
AR : pituitary, thyroid gland, adrenal glands, lymphatics.
   Particular care must be taken in treatment of a pregnant woman especially in the first three months of a first pregnancy or where there has been a previous miscarriage.

(b) *Male problems:* the most common problems associated with these glands include *infertility* and *prostate problems*, the latter affecting many men in later life.

DR : testes, prostate.
AR : pituitary, thyroid gland, adrenal glands, lymphatics and
     bladder, ureter tubes and kidneys (with prostate
     problems).

4. The Respiratory System

Asthma: in this condition breathing difficulties are experienced
on exhaling and there may be bouts of wheezing and coughing.
It can be caused by an allergic condition or may be due to
tension and stress.
DR : lungs, bronchi.
AR : solar plexus, cervical and thoracic spine, adrenal glands,
     ileo-caecal valve, pituitary, thyroid gland and repro-
     ductive glands, heart.

Bronchitis: breathing difficulties occur in this disorder where
there is inflammation of the lining of the bronchial tubes of the
lungs. A persistent cough is usually present.
DR : lungs, bronchi.
AR : solar plexus, lymphatics, ileo-caecal valve, adrenal
     glands.

Emphysema: with this condition there is a loss of elasticity of the
lung tissue which prevents the normal 'spring back' of the tissue
on expiration. Breathing difficulties thus occur when breathing
out and other symptoms will include a shortness of breath and a
cough.
DR : lungs, bronchi.
AR : solar plexus, adrenal glands, ileo-caecal valve.

5. The Heart and Circulatory System

All heart conditions must be treated with extreme care so as not
to over-stimulate the heart.
Angina: with angina there is an insufficient blood supply to the
heart muscles which can result in a short, sharp pain being
experienced in the heart area of the chest. The pain may also
extend up towards the shoulder and possibly down the left arm.
The symptoms are very similar to those of a heart attack, but
not as serious.

DR : heart.

AR : solar plexus, adrenal glands, shoulder and arm (if pain in these areas).

High blood pressure (Hypertension): blood pressure is the pressure exerted by the blood on the vessel walls and when it is raised this puts an extra strain on the heart and the blood vessels. The causes of high blood pressure are many and may involve stress, dietary factors, glandular imbalances and faulty elimination. The symptoms which result include headaches, dizziness, noises in the ears and pains in the chest.

DR : heart.

AR : solar plexus, adrenal glands, kidneys, big toe areas.

Circulatory problems: the overall general massage of all the reflex areas in the feet will greatly improve the blood circulation of all parts of the body. *Chilblains* affecting the hands, and feet can often be helped. Varicose veins once present, however, may be difficult to clear, though the treatment should help to prevent worsening of the condition and also help to prevent further varicose veins from forming.

DR : heart, direct massage to zone related areas.

AR : intestines, liver.

Conditions of thrombosis and phlebitis would normally not be treated with reflexology.

6.   The Lymphatic System

Since the system helps fight infection in the body, the reflexes to the lymphatics will be important in any condition where there is infection. In particular, the reflexes to the lymph nodes associated with the area affected will be important. The spleen reflex must also be remembered in infections, since the spleen is a part of the lymphatic system.

Breast lumps: these are often due to blocked lymph nodes in the breast and are not necessarily malignant.

DR : breast.

AR : pituitary, muscles of chest and arm (following removal of a breast).

Throat infections
DR : throat.
AR : neck, upper lymph nodes.

Shingles: this is a condition where a virus, similar to the chicken pox virus, affects the peripheral nerves causing their inflammation with great pain in certain areas. The sites most commonly affected are the chest and face, including the eyes, and a cluster of blisters develops on the skin over the area of the nerve affected. Following an attack of shingles, the pain may persist in the area affected for a considerable time after the blistering has subsided.
DR : reflex relating to area affected.
AR : lymphatics, spleen, solar plexus.

7. The Digestive System
Heartburn: this is not, in fact, caused by the heart and the sharp burning feeling experienced in the chest is due to the painful contraction of the muscles of the oesophagus contracting when the acid contents of the stomach flow back into the oesophagus.
DR : oesophagus, chest region.
AR : stomach, solar plexus, adrenal glands.

Indigestion (Dyspepsia): this may be caused by nervousness, stress and the wrong foods.
DR : stomach.
AR : solar plexus, diaphragm.

Hiatus hernia: a hernia refers to a condition where there is an abnormal protrusion of an organ through an opening in its surrounding structures, and a hiatus hernia refers to the protrusion of the stomach through the oesophageal opening in the diaphragm. This can result in pain being experienced along with indigestion and sometimes difficulty in swallowing.
DR : stomach.
AR : diaphragm, solar plexus, adrenal glands.

Ulcers: an ulcer is an open sore in a body surface and the most common sites are the stomach (gastric ulcer) and the small intestine (duodenal ulcer). An ulcer may result from poor diet or stress.

DR : stomach (gastric), duodenum (duodenal).

AR : solar plexus, diaphragm, adrenal glands.

Constipation: with constipation the bowel movements become irregular and in addition to the discomfort felt, if persistent, constipation can be a fore-runner of other disorders. These may involve the sinuses, the heart, varicose veins and ulcers on the leg, so it is most important for the bowel problem to be righted. Often dietary adjustments will normalize bowel movements but reflexology can help to improve the muscle movements of the large intestine.

DR : large intestine (particularly in the sigmoid colon, splenic flexure and hepatic flexure), ileo-caecal valve.

AR : small intestine, liver, gall bladder, solar plexus, adrenal glands, lower spine.

Flatulence (wind): in this case part of the digestive tract becomes distended with gas which escapes either upwards, if in the stomach, or downwards, if in the large intestine. It can be associated with eating the wrong foods and stress, particularly when eating.

DR : stomach, large intestine, ileo-caecal valve.

AR : solar plexus, diaphragm, liver, gall bladder, small intestine.

Colitis: this involves inflammation of the large intestine (colon) and may cause pain in the abdomen with constipation and diarrhoea.

DR : large intestine.

AR : solar plexus, adrenal glands.

Haemorrhoids: these are varicose veins in the region of the rectum and can result from persistent constipation.

DR : rectum.

AR : large intestine (particularly sigmoid colon), solar plexus, adrenal glands.

Hepatitis: in this condition the liver becomes inflamed due to a virus infection. Jaundice often results.

DR : liver.

AR : lymphatics, spleen, gall bladder, kidneys, pituitary.

Gall stones: in this painful condition stones consisting of mainly cholesterol and bile pigments settle in the gall bladder. It is possible, provided the stones are not too large, for them to be passed down the bile duct into the small intestine from where they can be expelled from the body.

DR : gall bladder.

AR : bile duct, liver, solar plexus, adrenal glands.

Allergies: with food allergies, parts of the digestive tract have become oversensitive to certain substances and an allergy results. Reflexology may help to lessen the sensitivity and thus reduce the allergic response.

DR : digestive tract.

AR : adrenal glands, pituitary, spleen.

8.   The Urinary System

Kidney disorders: if the filtering systems of the kidneys, the nephrons, become infected then the condition of *nephritis* occurs. It is characterized by the presence of protein in the urine. *Stones* can also form in the kidney and if small may be passed unnoticed. If larger stones are formed they can become lodged in the neck of the kidney or in the ureter tube causing extreme pain. It is sometimes possible to help stones to be passed using reflexology. Variations in the amount of urine passed and its colour and odour may also indicate kidney disorders, though normal variations can occur due to diet and fluids taken.

DR : kidneys, ureter tubes, bladder.

AR : lymphatics (if infection), adrenal glands, pituitary, solar plexus.

Bladder disorders: infection and inflammation of the bladder can occur which produce a burning sensation when passing urine;

this condition is known as *cystitis*. With *incontinence*, the muscles of the bladder have become weak and nervous factors may also be involved. An enlarged prostate gland in males may affect the bladder, as may pregnancy in women.

DR : bladder, ureter tubes, kidneys.

AR : lymphatics (if infection), adrenal glands, pituitary, prostate.

9. The Skin

Skin disorders: the many different disorders which affect the skin can often be helped by reflexology and these include such conditions as *eczema, psoriasis, dermatitis, acne* and miscellaneous *rashes*. Some skin conditions may be a direct allergy to a substance and also dietary adjustments can often be helpful to skin problems. In many cases a stress and tension factor may also be involved.

DR : reflex area corresponding to body part covered by affected area of skin.

AR : kidneys, adrenal glands, thyroid gland, pituitary, solar plexus, intestines, lymphatics (if infection).

A wide variety of conditions have been discussed with a description of how reflexology treatment can be applied to them. The specific treatment of cancer has not been mentioned but reflexology can be of benefit in this area. Even if it cannot bring about complete recovery, the overall balancing effect will help to strengthen the whole body to help fight the condition, with the relaxation induced by the treatment helping the patient to cope better both mentally and physically. There are obviously many more conditions not mentioned which may well be helped, and similar treatment procedures will be followed to help remove or alleviate them.

Chapter 6

Case Histories

Having seen in theory how reflexology can help a wide variety of conditions, it is probably helpful to potential patients to read of true case histories. The following are reports of treatment given either by the author or students who have trained with her and help to verify the effects which reflexology can have. As in previous chapters, the conditions will be described under the various systems of the body relating primarily to the most troublesome symptom for which the patient sought help. In many of these cases, other symptoms were also involved and helped and, although it must be stressed that reflexology treats the person as a whole, looking at the various disorders affecting the different systems allows a convenient way of discussing the conditions which may be benefit.

1. The Head

Migraine
Numerous different examples of successful treatment of this condition could be cited and it does seem that headaches and migraine are particularly helped by reflexology, possibly due to its relaxing effect.

A lady aged forty-six had suffered with migraines for about fifteen years. Initially they used to occur about ten days before her period but gradually became more frequent. The pain usually affected the left side of the head and was accompanied by sickness. This lady had been told by her doctor that she had a hormonal imbalance which had persisted following the birth of her second child. She also suffered with sinus trouble. At the first treatment session the feet appeared to be rather stiff and many of the reflex areas showed tenderness, including the reflexes to the pituitary top of the head, the neck, sinuses, eyes, shoulders, lower spine, thyroid, liver, bladder, kidneys, adrenals, ovaries, uterus and solar plexus. As regular treatment sessions followed, the reflex areas became less tender though the areas relating to the head, neck, sinuses, eyes and solar plexus still showed some tenderness. This lady found that the frequency of her migraines decreased and after about eight sessions the migraines did not occur unless she had put herself under particular stress. The migraines were, however, less severe and if they did develop, they passed off more quickly. Since this lady did seem to lead a very busy life looking after her family and various elderly relatives, in addition to working part-time, it was recommended that treatment be continued at intervals of six weeks to help keep the body more balanced. This course of action was followed to great benefit. Migraines still occurred but only when the lady pushed herself too far — a signal being sent out from the body to slow down! In general, the lady was less tense and fitter and was also more aware when she was becoming too tense. She could thus recognize the warning signs and prevent a migraine from occurring.

*   *   *

A lady aged thirty-six had experienced migraines for twenty years. At one time she had had one weekly but when she came for treatment the condition did not appear regularly. The very bad headaches could last for up to four days. Several items had been cut out of the diet in case they were causing her complaint. At the first treatment session, the feet were not particularly sensitive and a slight reaction was found from the reflexes to the pituitary, head, eyes, neck, spine, kidneys, adrenals, hips and knees. In the week after the treatment the lady had an upset stomach and the symptoms of a cold — both possible signs of a form of healing crisis. At the next treatment one week later, the feet showed more tender reflexes than before with the liver, gall bladder and digestive tract areas reacting. After eight weekly treatment sessions, this lady was no longer developing migraines and although on a few occasions she had felt as if she was going to have a migraine this had not developed. Some reflex areas in the feet still responded as tendernesses but in general the body had become more balanced.

Stroke

A lady in her seventies requested treatment having suffered a stroke four years previously which had left her paralysed on her left side. She wore a caliper on her left leg and the left arm could not be moved away from the side of her body. The following areas in the feet were found to be tender — pituitary, head, face, spine, ears, stomach, large intestine, spleen, kidneys, adrenals, sciatic nerve. When the areas were massaged in the paralysed left foot, a jerking reaction occurred. At the second treatment session similar areas showed tenderness, including the reflex areas to the shoulder, arm and neck. As treatment progressed a degree of feeling returned to the leg. After fifteen treatments it became possible to move the left arm away from the body and straighten it and the lady could move the left arm slightly herself. Treatments continued for a period during which time the lady found she was able to walk slightly better and the arm became much freer.

Parkinson's disease

A lady in her seventies had been diagnosed as having Parkinson's disease one year prior to trying reflexology treatment, though probably the condition had been present for longer. The symptoms started with trembling in the right leg and had then developed to give trembling in the hands, with rigidity of the muscles and slow movement. On walking in the morning the rigidity was very bad and there was also a great deal of pain throughout the body which eased slightly as the day went on. Before this condition developed the lady had always had good health. At the first treatment session the feet were extremely sensitive to the massage and a very careful treatment was required. Most of the reflex areas were found to be tender and the feet and ankles were stiff. This lady's husband was most interested to learn how to give the treatment to help his wife and was aware that many treatments would be required before results became evident. Nine treatment sessions were given at fortnightly intervals due to the distance which the elderly couple had to travel for treatment, and in the week between the husband gave his wife a treatment. Although after this time the disorder was still present, the lady reported that she was feeling better in herself and was able to get more tasks done in the day. Her daughter who had not seen her for several months since she lived abroad had said that her mother looked brighter in the face and able to do more. In this case, even though the condition had not disappeared, there had been an improvement and certainly no deterioration and the lady's husband was to continue giving regular treatment.

Multiple sclerosis

A lady had had multiple sclerosis for eight years and the right arm was immobile, there was swelling in the abdomen with incontinence, a prolapsed rectum, difficulty with swallowing and a weight problem. After two treatments the swelling in the abdomen had reduced and the passing of water became controlled. With progressive treatments the body became more balanced with a reduction in symptoms and the lady continued with treatments at regular intervals for a period of about one year since she found it so beneficial.

Sinus problems

A young lady in her twenties had developed a sinus problem about one year before commencing treatment. She felt worse in the mornings when the nose would be blocked, her eyes would water and she would have a headache. Blowing the nose, often caused it to bleed. In addition, this lady was prone to ear infections and in the past had had bronchial trouble. At the first treatment session the feet were quite sensitive, with tender reflexes being found in the areas relating to the head, face, neck, sinuses, Eustachian tube, eyes, liver, gall bladder, intestines, ileo-caecal valve, kidneys, adrenals, solar plexus, heart, ovaries and uterus. The lady felt very relaxed by the end of the treatment and also felt that her sinuses were clearer. At the second treatment session she reported that she had felt tired after treatment but during the week her sinuses had felt much better. Treatment continued for a six week period during which time the sinus problem cleared and the lady felt much better in herself and more energetic. At the time of her period she had not experienced the normal pain which lasted for the first two days of the menstrual flow and also her period had occurred after four weeks instead of six weeks or more. She also reported that she was sleeping better, had lost weight and was able to concentrate for longer periods. After six treatments the reflexes in the feet were considerably less sensitive but there was still a slight feeling of 'grittiness' evident in the sinus areas.

Eye disorders

A lady in her sixties had developed dry eyes for the past two years following a bad attack of conjunctivitis and had to use drops in her eyes. The first treatment session showed tender reflex areas to the pituitary, neck, spine, shoulder, eyes, sinuses, kidneys and adrenals. At the second treatment session the lady said that she had not used her eye drops at all since the first treatment and that the eyes were again producing tears — she was amazed and delighted! Treatment continued for seven weeks during which time the eyes caused no more problems and the general health of the lady also improved.

*   *   *

A lady receiving treatment for a foot problem found that as a result of a course of treatment not only did the foot problem ease but her eyesight also improved and she needed to wear her glasses on very few occasions.

Ear disorders

A man had suffered with tinnitus for about seven years and had deafness in the right ear. At the first treatment the reflex areas to the pituitary, neck, ears, Eustachian tubes, sinuses, lungs, spine, kidneys and adrenals all showed tenderness. The patient's feet were rather tense. On the second visit the man said that during the week he had coughed a lot and brought up mucus but the ears were no different. During the second treatment, when the feet again showed several tender areas, the pulsation in the ears increased. On the third visit the patient said that he had been feeling better but was still coughing. After nine treatments, the patient reported that the noises had ceased in the ears and the coughing had also stopped. It appeared that the noises in the ears may have been connected with mucus congestion of the sinuses and lungs which when cleared had eased the ear problem. The hearing had not improved but had been caused by injury to the ear.

*   *   *

Another tinnitus sufferer, a lady in her fifties, found that regular treatment controlled the noises in her ear and helped relax her, especially by reducing the tension which she usually experienced in her head and neck.

2.   The Musculo-Skeletal System

Spinal problems

So many people suffer from back problems at some time in their life and numerous case histories could be written of where help has been given. A gentleman in his fifties decided to try reflexology treatment having had back problems for many years. The pain experienced was usually on the right side in the mid-back but could also occur lower down the back with pain in the buttock and leg. At the first treatment this gentleman could not stand erect due to the pain and muscle spasm in his back. Treatment was emphasized on the reflexes to the spine, hips,

sacro-iliac joints and adrenals and by the end of the treatment
the man was able to stand up straight and walk out of the
treatment room free of pain. Treatment was continued for eight
weeks, during which time the back problem did not return.
This man returned for treatment at intervals whenever he felt
twinges of pain returning in his back and one or two treatments
were able to right the problem on each occasion.

Fibrositis in the neck
A lady in her thirties had suffered with fibrositis in her neck for
five years when she first came for treatment. Mainly the right
side of her neck was affected and this caused pain across the
right shoulder blade, in the right shoulder and also sometimes
down the right arm. At the first treatment the reflex areas to the
head, neck, shoulder, shoulder girdle, arm, cervical spine and
solar plexus were all tender. On rotating the big toe joints these
were found to be extremely stiff. At the next treatment session
one week later, the lady reported that the pain had lessened
considerably and her neck felt much freer. After four treatments
the pain had cleared except for one instance of slight discomfort
resulting when driving a car. This lady was also recommended
to do exercises for her neck to keep this area as relaxed as
possible.

Golfer's elbow
An international sports player developed golfer's elbow which
caused great pain in the elbow when playing both squash and
tennis. Since the person involved played both these sports
professionally a quick recovery was essential. The reflex areas
in the feet were not particularly tender since the lady was quite
fit and healthy, apart from the elbow problem and a slight knee
and lower back problem. The tender areas were the reflexes to
the neck, shoulder, arm, knee, spine and solar plexus, kidneys
and adrenals. After the first treatment the pain had eased and
after four treatments the arm and elbow could be moved
normally. The lady was so impressed with the treatment that
she has continued with regular treatment sessions at monthly

intervals to help prevent further injury to the joints and also to help the knee and back problems which are aggravated at times but respond well to the treatment.

Sciatica

A young gentleman in his thirties sought help for a back problem which had kept him off work for three months. Injury had initially occurred following the lifting of a heavy object which had strained the lower back, causing pain in this area and also sciatica with the nerve pain extending from the lower back across the buttock and down the back of the leg to the knee. At the first treatment session the feet appeared to be quite stiff with tender reflex areas relating to the pituitary, neck, sinuses, solar plexus, kidneys, adrenals, lower back, sciatic areas, hips, sacro-iliac joints and muscles of the buttock. After the third treatment the patient reported that he had been able to cut down on the number of pain-killers which he had been taking and after the fourth treatment was able to manage without any. Following eight treatment sessions, the patient felt well enough to return to work but was warned to avoid any heavy lifting. The sciatic pain had cleared and he had also noticed an improvement in his sinus condition. This gentleman returns for treatment at intervals when he begins to feel pain in his back again; this occurs if he puts the back under extra strain and the treatment is able to right the condition often with only two or three treatments.

Arthritis

A gentleman in his seventies was waiting to have a hip replacement operation following the development of arthritis in his right hip. He was hoping that the reflexology treatment would ease the pain which he was feeling. The reflex areas in the feet to the pituitary, head, neck, eyes, ears, Eustachian tube, solar plexus, parathyroids, hips, sacro-iliac joints, kidneys and adrenals were all fairly sensitive at the first treatment session. After the first treatment the patient reported less pain in the hip and this improvement continued with further treatments. A course of four treatments was followed and the gentleman improved so much that his specialist decided against an operation on the hip. The gentleman also found that his prostate problem improved with treatment and he needed to get up less frequently in the night to visit the bathroom.

*   *   *

A lady in her sixties was having problems with her feet and had been told that arthritis had developed in the joints between the phalanges and the metatarsals. In the past she had had operations on her feet for various reasons and was now finding considerable discomfort when walking. After a course of ten treatments this lady found that her feet had become much more comfortable and had also found an improvement in both her neck which had become stiff and her eyes which tended to be tired and watery.

Knee problem

A young gentleman had injured his knee in a road accident. This had left him with a pain in the knee below the knee cap. The pain was intermittent, but restricting, and sometimes the knee would lock. At the first treatment session the man was worried that his feet would not be able to be touched since he was very ticklish but in fact, he found the treatment very pleasant and relaxing. Several areas of the feet showed tender reflexes including those to the pituitary, neck, sinuses, Eustachian tube, eyes, liver, spine, knees, kidneys and adrenals. During the first treatment he felt his sinuses becoming unblocked and experienced a popping sensation in his ears. After the first treatment the man felt no further pain in his knee and also found that his sinus problem had cleared. Two further treatments were given and the problems did not return.

Gout

A gentleman in his sixties came for reflexology treatment for a skin complaint for which regular treatment was given. He was also a sufferer of gout but since receiving a course of reflexology this condition has not troubled him.

3.   The Endocrine System

Thyroid problems
A lady aged fifty-two had for three weeks felt pain in the back of the head and neck and for six weeks had had a swelling of the thyroid gland which was very sore to touch. At the first treatment session the feet were rather tense and tender areas were found in the reflex areas to the pituitary, head, neck, thyroid, ears, solar plexus, stomach, intestines, kidneys, adrenals, uterus and ovaries. By the end of the treatment the lady felt very relaxed. At the second visit she reported that she had had a bad headache for two days after the treatment but that this had then cleared and her thyroid gland was less swollen. By the third treatment the thyroid gland was noticeably less swollen and was not sore to touch. This lady received five treatments and then ceased treatment since she considered her condition to have been cleared.

*   *   *

A lady in her fifties had had a partial removal of her thyroid gland in her thirties and had had no further problems until about six years prior to seeking treatment when the gland had become overactive again and caused her eyes to protrude. She was also feeling tired and had gained weight. There was also swelling of the ankles. The first treatment session showed tender reflex areas to the pituitary, head, face, neck, sinuses, eyes, thyroid, liver, stomach, solar plexus, kidneys, adrenals and lymphatics. At the second session the lady reported that the treatment had made her feel very tired but that the pressure behind the eyes had reduced and the eyes were less protruding. The ankles were less swollen as well. Regular treatment continued to show improvement of the condition apart from a set-back for a few weeks when the patient had a bad bout of flu.

This lady continued with the treatment for several months as she found it helpful and, apart from helping the thyroid condition, it was enabling her to cope better with a particularly difficult time she was having at work.

Diabetes

A retired gentleman developed aching legs and feet and was eventually found to have diabetes. The condition had only been diagnosed for a couple of months when reflexology treatment was commenced. For the first three treatment sessions very little tenderness was felt at the reflex areas in the feet and the feet were cold, with much hard skin present. From the fourth treatment more sensitivity appeared, particularly in the reflexes to the pituitary, liver, pancreas, solar plexus, kidneys and adrenals. The patient began to feel better with less pain in the feet and legs. At the eighth treatment the patient said that he had been cleared by the hospital diabetic clinic and told that further visits were no longer necessary. Two more reflexology treatments were given and the gentleman continued in fairly good health with no sign of the diabetes returning. He was also careful with his diet.

Female problems

A young lady in her twenties had an hormonal imbalance which caused irregular periods and a poor skin. She had also had problems with infections of the uterus. The first treatment session showed tender reflex areas of the pituitary, face, spine, thyroid, solar plexus, kidneys, adrenals, ovaries, uterus and lymphatics. The lady said that she felt wonderful after the treatment and had enjoyed having her feet massaged. At the second treatment she said that she had been feeling much better and although she had had bad pain the evening before her period had started this had passed off by the next day, when usually it lasted for a couple of days. Similar reflex areas showed tenderness and as treatment progressed the lady continued to feel better and also showed an improvement in the condition of her skin. Twelve treatments were given.

*   *   *

A young lady of thirty came for treatment to help with postnatal depression from which she was suffering after the birth of her son. She was on anti-depressant tablets and felt generally unwell. At the first treatment session the feet did not show many tender reflex areas though there was a slight reaction to massage to the reflexes to the pituitary, head, eyes, liver, gall bladder, intestines, solar plexus, uterus, kidneys and adrenals. At the second treatment session, the lady seemed very depressed and was no better. The feet were, however, slightly more sensitive. At the third treatment, the patient reported that she had had a much better week and was feeling brighter. Treatment continued for six weeks during which time a marked improvement in the depression occurred and the lady found herself once more able to cope with things.

*   *   *

A lady who was twelve weeks pregnant was troubled with sickness which had also occurred in her two previous pregnancies and lasted from the third month through to the time she gave birth. There was not just a feeling of nausea but she was actually sick at least six times a day. At the first treatment, although the lady seemed relaxed, tender reflex areas were found for the pituitary, neck, eyes, liver, stomach, intestines, uterus and spine. At the second visit she was delighted to report that the sickness had been reduced. The feet still showed tender areas and regular treatment was given for six weeks by which time she was experiencing only feelings of nausea but no actual sickness.

4.   The Respiratory System

Asthma
A lady in her sixties had had asthma for four years when first

coming for reflexology treatment. Before this she had been a very active healthy person and there seemed no obvious reason for the development of the asthma. The reflexes in the feet were not particularly sensitive but there was a slight reaction in the areas of the pituitary, head, face, neck, lungs, kidneys and adrenals. As a course of treatment progressed, the feet never appeared to show many tender reflexes but the condition gradually improved. After twelve sessions the lady felt clear of her symptoms and was able to walk as normal without becoming breathless or wheezy.

*   *   *

A boy of sixteen had been troubled since the age of seven with asthma and hay fever. He had tried different diets and treatments to help the condition, with limited success. At the first treatment the feet showed many tender reflexes, including those to the pituitary, neck, spine, sinuses, eyes, lungs, solar plexus, large intestines, kidneys and adrenals. The feet also perspired a great deal. By the second treatment the symptoms had eased, though the boy still sounded rather nasal. The feet were perspiring less. After five treatments there was little nasal congestion and no wheeziness in the chest and the boy was feeling much better.

Emphysema

A lady in her sixties had emphysema. This had developed more in the past four to five years and left her very breathless after any slight exertion. During treatment the feet were found to be extremely sensitive and only a very light pressure could be applied, with many reflexes showing tenderness. After the treatment the lady experienced a tingling sensation throughout her body. The first treatment caused a considerable improvement of the condition and she was able to walk further without getting out of breath and also walk upstairs. This improvement continued but a course of ten treatments did not clear the condition completely. This lady did, however, smoke which was obviously aggravating the condition and preventing a complete recovery.

Bronchitis
A young boy of six was continually off school because of bronchitis, sinus trouble and bad coughs. A course of seven treatments were given during which time the boy only missed one day at school due to a stomach upset. He did not develop any cold or cough and had no further reoccurrence of bronchitis. His parents reported that he was also eating well, which had been a problem previously.

5.   The Heart and Circulatory System

Angina
A retired lady had suffered a heart attack which had been followed by intermittent attacks of angina. This lady also suffered with asthma and constipation. At the first treatment the feet showed several tender reflex areas including the reflexes to the pituitary, neck, eyes, shoulders, lungs, heart, thyroid, solar plexus, liver, intestines, ileo-caecal valve, kidneys and adrenals. At the second treatment session the lady appeared to be very breathless and the feet were very sensitive. At the third treatment she was able to report an improvement in her constipation, less breathlessness and less pain from her angina. By the end of the treatment session, the lady was looking much better in herself. Treatments continued for twelve weeks and the symptoms all showed improvement.

High blood-pressure
A gentleman in his seventies considered himself reasonably fit for his age, apart from the fact that he had been told he had high blood-pressure. A course of five treatments at somewhat irregular intervals helped this gentleman to become more relaxed and balanced with the resultant normalizing of his blood pressure — much to the surprise of his doctor!

Poor circulation

A lady in her twenties had had poor circulation in the fingers
since the age of about nine. This caused the hands to be cold
with swelling of the fingers and redness of the hands and
fingers. Although the symptoms were far worse in the winter
months, the problem still persisted when the weather was
warmer. With a short course of treatment the swelling in the
fingers reduced even though it was winter. The hands also felt
warmer though the redness persisted.

Heart attack and thrombosis

An elderly lady had suffered these two conditions four years
prior to her receiving treatment. This had left her in a poor
physical state and had become virtually bed-ridden and had not
been out of her house for two years. On first treatment of the
feet there was little response but on subsequent treatments more
feeling became apparent. Many reflex areas were tender but the
lady began to feel better in herself and began to walk in her
house for short periods. After five treatments she went for a
short walk in the street where she lived and was delighted with
the improvement. Even after a course of treatment had
finished, her condition continued to improve and she reported
that she had walked to the nearby shops and caught a bus to
visit her sister — something she thought she would never be
doing again.

6. The Lymphatic System

Ear and throat infections

A young lady in her thirties was troubled by persistent ear and
throat infections and was generally in a 'run-down' state. She
also suffered with headaches, a slight sinus problem and pain
before her periods. Regular treatment sessions helped improve
the body's resistance to infections and these occurred much less
frequently. Although this lady still showed some reoccurrence
of her symptoms through overwork, her general health
improved after about eight treatment sessions. Treatment was

continued at monthly periods to help maintain the balance in the body.

Shingles

A man in his thirties developed shingles after being in contact with someone who had chicken pox. Blisters were present around the front and back at waist level. This area was extremely painful and felt as if the skin was being stretched. This gentleman came for treatment the day after he was found to have shingles but the reflex areas in the feet were not too sensitive to touch. One treatment produced a significant improvement and the man stopped taking the pain-killers he had been prescribed. After one week he was considerably better and after three treatments no symptoms were present and the man felt well again.

7. The Digestive System

Duodenal ulcer

A gentleman aged forty had had stomach problems since the age of ten. In later years he had become more aware of his diet and was careful about the foods he ate but had developed a duodenal ulcer which caused him pain. At the first treatment session the feet were rather tense and did not show many tender reflex areas. At the second treatment the feet were less tense and more responsive, with tender reflexes to the pituitary, sinuses, stomach, small and large intestines, solar plexus, spine and adrenals. After four treatment sessions, the gentleman reported that he had had no further pain from his ulcer. He continued to follow a careful diet.

Constipation

A middle-aged lady was suffering much discomfort in the abdomen due to constipation. She also suffered from flatulence. In addition she had catarrh and painful varicose veins in her legs. When first receiving treatment the lady appeared very tense and the feet showed many tender reflex areas, including those to the pituitary, head, sinuses, neck, eyes, liver, stomach, small intestine, large intestine, rectum, heart and solar plexus. At the second treatment the lady seemed much brighter and found an improvement in her catarrh. Her bowel movements had also been slightly more regular. Six treatments were given, by which time the digestive problems and catarrh were greatly improved, though there was still pain associated with the varicose veins in the legs.

Irritable bowel

A young lady had developed an irritable bowel, along with other symptoms, following the birth of her daughter three years prior to first receiving reflexology treatment. At the first treatment session the feet were not very sensitive but at the second visit the lady reported that her bowel movements had been more normal and the pain in her abdomen was less. After six treatments the lady found a great improvement in her health with fewer headaches, less fluid retention and more regular bowel movements. She was also much more relaxed.

Hepatitis

A young gentleman developed jaundice following an attack of hepatitis. After three treatments the yellow colour to his skin had disappeared, though the reflex areas to the liver, spleen and stomach were still extremely tender. He felt less tired and his blood count had improved considerably. Further treatments helped to accelerate the recovery from this condition.

8. The Urinary System

Kidney disorders

A middle aged lady had kidney failure and was in a very weak physical state but unwilling to receive conventional medical treatment. A course of four reflexology treatments caused an improvement in the functioning of the kidneys, with more colour to the urine. The treatment also helped the lady's constipation and gave her more energy. Unfortunately this lady had to discontinue with treatment due to moving away from the area, so further results were not known.

Water retention

A gentleman in his forties was suffering with water retention accompanied by sharp pains in the urethra. There was also a frequent desire to pass water but an inability to do so. The reflexes in this case were very sensitive at the first treatment, particularly those areas relating to the pituitary, spine, eyes, solar plexus, bladder, ureter tubes, kidneys, adrenals, prostate and testes. After five treatments the gentleman found an improvement in the condition except for one or two bad days; the pain disappeared and the passing of water became normal.

Bladder weakness

A gentleman in his forties sought help for a problem of leakage from the bladder. He experienced no pain or frequent desire to pass water but was worried that the problem might develop. At the first treatment the feet showed many tender reflex areas including those to the pituitary, neck, eyes, thyroid, bladder, kidneys, adrenals, prostate, testes and lymphatics. A slight improvement was noticed after the first treatment and this improvement increased with subsequent treatments. After seven treatments the man considered that his problem had been righted.

9.   The Skin

Eczema

A young child of three had dry eczema on the face, behind the ears, on the neck, arms and legs. This caused her to scratch the skin, which was raw in places. The child also had a tendency towards asthma if she caught a cold. At the first treatment the child behaved very well and allowed the feet to be worked on without any fuss. At the second treatment the skin of the face looked greatly improved and the child's mother said that the little girl had been sleeping better. After seven treatments the skin was showing an overall improvement with far less irritation and thus less scratching of the skin.

Urticaria

A gentleman in his thirties had for three years suffered with a form of urticaria which caused large red wheals to appear on the skin over most of the body. The skin also looked red and inflamed. Apart from the skin problem the man was quite healthy. At the first treatment session many reflex areas in the feet were sensitive, including those to the pituitary, head, face, liver, stomach, intestines, solar plexus, heart, kidneys and adrenals. Following treatment, wheals appeared on the skin of the feet but disappeared after about ten minutes. After the first treatment the gentleman reported that he had managed without taking any anti-histamine tablets for most of the time. A course of six treatments was given, during which time the redness of the skin became greatly reduced. Irritation of the skin also lessened, and the patient rarely needed to take anti-histamine tablets. The man found that if a skin reaction did occur, it went within about fifteen minutes. This man's condition was also aided by improvements to his diet.

Face rash

A teenage girl developed a rash on her face. This started with irritation and then became dry and inflamed but without the appearance of any nodules under the skin or weeping. The problem had been present for a year when the girl came for treatment. The first treatment showed tender reflex areas for the pituitary, head, face, neck, thyroid, solar plexus, liver, intestines, kidneys, adrenals and lymphatics. After one month the rash had disappeared and the girl was feeling relaxed and well.

The case histories which have been described are but a few of the very many which could have been mentioned. They will, it is hoped, indicate how the treatment can so often be of help. Not all of the cases mentioned showed a complete removal of the symptoms but in each case there was a considerable improvement.

Chapter 7

Reflexology as a Preventative Therapy

The preceding chapters explain how reflexology can be of help in the treatment of various disorders. In general, people tend to wait until ill-health develops before seeking help to try and right the disorder, either by conventional means or by one of the alternative therapies. Often a quick recovery is expected even though the problem may have been developing for a considerable length of time. In the first instance most people start life with a potential for good health, and illness or disease only results from abuse of the body through such factors as diet, stress and the lifestyle followed. Problems such as allergies and viruses occur when the body is not strong enough to overcome them and it is usually found that people develop a weakness in one of the eliminating systems such as the lungs, skin, kidneys, or digestive system which results in that system not functioning correctly, either continuously or from time to time. Reflexology treatment can be of help in trying to strengthen these weaknesses and thus prevent the symptoms occurring so frequently.

There is now, however, a growing trend towards caring for the whole self more constantly in order to reduce the likelihood of being ill. This caring is not only for the physical body by, for example, eating more sensibly but also for the mind by, for example, relaxation techniques. Reflexology can be of great benefit as a preventative therapy and offers a means of caring for the whole self. By having treatments at regular intervals, the body can be maintained in a more balanced state with resulting continued good health. The intervals between treatments can vary from person to person and may involve weeks or months. In addition, the diagnostic capability of reflexology can be employed, enabling possible imbalances in the body from becoming troublesome symptoms. The fact that the reflex areas in the feet appear tender when massaged if the corresponding body area is out of balance can indicate which parts of the body are not working as well as they might. Since the method is a very sensitive one, it is possible to detect imbalances in the early stages and thus prevent more serious imbalances from resulting. The overall relaxing effect of the treatment can also be of great benefit in preventing imbalances arising.

It is probably unrealistic to expect the majority of people to have perfect health throughout their life, especially since the decision to take more care of the body often develops following ill-health. In this respect it is often found that where a person has had a course of reflexology treatment for specific disorders which have been corrected, if similar or other disorders develop the treatment tends to be more quickly effective in helping to relieve or right the condition, especially if treatment is received shortly after the condition arises.

It has been emphasized that a full treatment involving massage of all the reflex areas in the feet is always administered and this really is the most beneficial way for treatment to be given. Also, for the best results, the treatment needs to be applied in the correct manner. Nevertheless, in some cases, it may be recommended by the practitioner that the patient tries to work on specific reflex areas him/herself between treatment sessions which may aid in the relief of isolated symptoms. This extra work acts as a boost to the treatment, though it must be remembered that it may not be reaching the cause of the problem but rather the result of the problem. Many people have been known to work on just a few reflex areas for the relief of minor problems such as headaches, toothache, constipation and tension. Some people may not find it that easy to work on the reflex areas in their own feet and in these instances it may be more convenient to work on the reflex areas found in the hands.

Hand Reflexology

As in the feet, reflex areas are found in the hands corresponding to all the parts of the body and again these are arranged in such a manner as to form a logical pattern of the body in the hands.

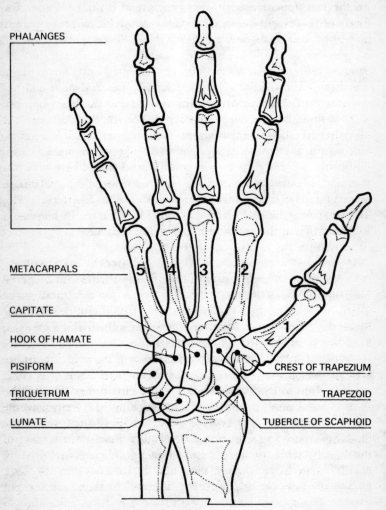

Figure 22. The bones of the hand.

Most of the reflex points are found in the palms, which can be considered the equivalent of the soles of the feet. The backs of the hands are equivalent to the tops of the feet and the five longitudinal zones described earlier are present in the hands, with each zone corresponding to the area below the digits. The bones of the hands are similarly arranged to the bones of the feet as can be seen by a description of the skeleton of the hand.

The structure of the hand

The bones of the fingers are called phalanges and each finger is composed of three phalanges, except for the thumb which has just two phalanges. The upper part of the hand below the phalanges consists of five metacarpal bones, each extending below one of the phalanges. The remainder of the bones in the hand are called carpal bones and the individual names of the bones are the scaphoid, lunate, triquetrum, pisiform, trapezoid, trapezium, capitate and hamate. (See Figure 22.) The bones are held in place and allowed a range of movements by various muscles, muscle tendons and ligaments.

The reflex areas of the hand

A less detailed description of the reflex areas in the hand will be given than for those reflex areas in the feet since the pattern of distribution of these areas is similar to that found in the feet. Since the hands are smaller than the feet, the reflex areas are found in smaller areas than in the feet and can also be slightly more difficult to detect precisely. However, the principle of the zones still exists in the hands and in whichever zone or zones a part is found in the body, the corresponding reflex area will be found in the same zone or zones of the hands. The transverse zones cannot be so easily applied to the hands since the phalanges and metacarpal bones occupy a substantial part of the hands, with the carpal bones occupying a comparatively smaller area in the hands than the tarsal bones in the feet. Imaginary lines corresponding to the waistline and diaphragm can be transposed onto the hands to act as a guide to the positioning of various reflexes. (See Figures 23 and 24.)

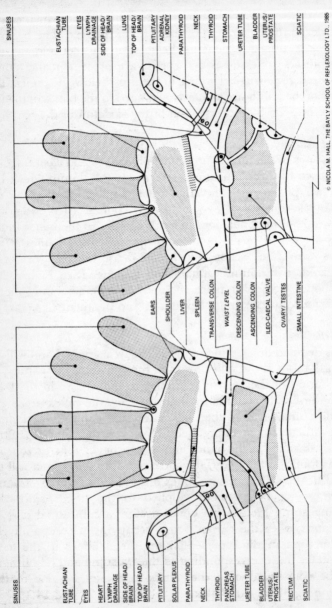

Figure 23. The reflexes of the palms of the hands.

© NICOLA M. HALL, THE BAYLY SCHOOL OF REFLEXOLOGY LTD., 1986

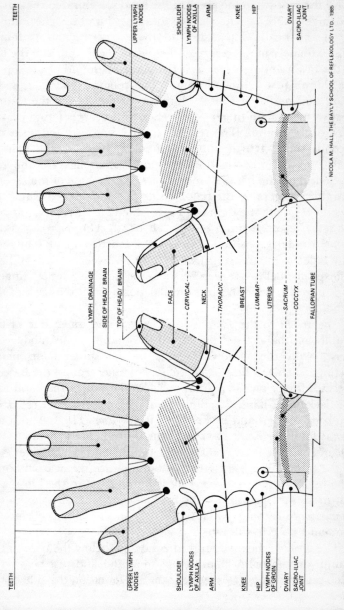

Figure 24. The reflexes of the backs of the hands.

All the reflexes to the areas of the head are found in regions of the fingers and, as with the big toes, the thumbs correspond to all of the head. The reflex to the *pituitary* gland is found approximately in the centre of the pad of the thumb and the top of the brain and *top of the head* reflex area is found at the top of the thumb just behind the nail. The reflex to the side of the brain and *side of the head* is found down the side of the thumb next to the second finger. The reflex to the *face* is found on the back of the thumb. The reflexes to the *sinuses* are found in the second, third, fourth and fifth fingers, both up the palmar surface of the fingers and up the sides. The reflexes to the *teeth* are found on the backs of the fingers. At the base of the second and third fingers on the palmar side of the hand are found the *eye* reflexes, with the right eye represented on the right hand and the left eye represented on the left hand. The *ear* reflexes are found similarly positioned below the fourth and fifth fingers. The reflex to the *Eustachian tube* is found between the eye and ear reflexes just below the web between the third and fourth fingers and may also be found in a similar position on the back of the hand.

The reflex to the *spine* is found down the inner side of the thumb and hand from the top of the thumb to just above the wrist, with the various regions of the spine again being distinguishable. The *shoulder* reflex is found around the base of the fifth finger on the palmar surface, the side of the hand and the back of the hand. Leading down from the shoulder reflex on the back of the hand is the reflex to the *arm*. The reflex to the *neck* is found around the base of the thumb. The reflexes to the *hip* and *knee* are found on the back of the hand on the outer side of the fifth zone close to the base of the fifth metacarpal bone. The reflex to the *sacro-iliac joint* is found close to the hip reflex but more in zone four on the back of the hand. A reflex to the *sciatic* nerve is found in all five zones on the palmar surface of the hand close to the wrist.

The *thyroid* reflex is found in zone one, below the base of the thumb on the palmar surface of the hand and just below the neck reflex. The *parathyroid* reflexes are found on the side of the thyroid reflex closest to zone two with an upper and lower reflex on both hands. The reflexes to the *adrenal* glands are found in zone two at about waist level of the palm of the hand just above the kidney reflexes. The reflex area to the *pancreas* is found in both left and right hands on the palmar surface in the area between the diaphragm and waist level in zones one, two and three on the left and zones one and two on the right. The reflexes to the reproductive glands are found on both the palmar surface and back of the hand just above the wrist with the *ovary* or *testes* reflex in zone five and the *uterus* or *prostate* reflex in zone one. The *Fallopian tube* reflex joins the ovary and uterus areas across the back of the hand.

The reflex area to the *lungs* is found on both the palmar surface and the back of both hands below the fingers and in the upper part of the hand above the level of the diaphragm. The *solar plexus* reflex is found in both hands on the palmar surface at diaphragm level in zones two and three.

The *heart* reflex, as in the feet, is found mainly in an area not quite corresponding with the zonal position of the heart in the body but in zones two and three of the palmar surface of the left hand, close to the lung area and above the level of the diaphragm.

The reflexes to the *lymphatic system* are found on the backs of the hands with the reflexes to the *upper lymph nodes* situated at the roots of the fingers, the *breast* reflexes situated in zones two, three and four above the waist level and the reflexes to the *lymph nodes of the groin* found across all five zones just above the wrist. The reflexes to the *lymph nodes of the axilla* are found just below the shoulder reflexes on the backs of the hands. The reflex to the *spleen* is found on the palmar surface of the left hand above the waist level in zones four and five. The reflex area to stimulate *lymph drainage* to the venous system in the neck is found in the web between the thumb and second finger on both the back and palm of both hands.

The *stomach* reflex is found on the palmar surface of both right and left hands mainly in zones one, two and three on the left and zone one on the right, above the waist level and below the diaphragm. The *oesophagus* reflex is in an area joining the stomach reflex from the neck area down the side of the ball of the thumb closest to zone two. The reflex area for the *small intestines* is found in the palms of both hands in zones one, two, three and four below the waist level and extending down to an area above the wrist. The large intestine is represented similarly in the hands as in the feet, with the *ileo-caecal valve* reflex on the palmar surface of the right hand in zones four and five a short distance above the wrist, with the *ascending colon* reflex leading up from this to about waist level and the *transverse colon* reflex leading from this across all five zones of the right hand and then all five zones of the left hand. The *descending colon* reflex leads downwards from the transverse colon reflex in the left hand in zones four and five before turning across towards zone one a short distance above the wrist with the reflex to the *sigmoid colon*. At the end of this reflex area in zone one is found the reflex to the *rectum*. As in the feet, the *liver* reflex is found predominantly in the right hand on the palmar surface in zones three, four and five between the diaphragm and waist level. The *gall bladder* reflex is found in zone three of the right hand just below the liver reflex.

The reflex to the *bladder* is found on both hands on the side and slightly to the back of the hand in zone one, close to the reflex to the lumbar region of the spine. A reflex for the *ureter tube* leads from the bladder area up to the *kidney* reflex, which is found on the palmar surface of both hands in zones two and three at approximately waist level.

It is usually found that the reflex areas in the hands are not so sensitive or tender as those areas in the feet and this may be partly due to the fact that the hands are constantly in use whereas the feet are for most of the time protected by the wearing of socks, stockings and shoes. The crystal deposits sometimes felt at reflex areas in the feet may also be felt in the hands. The reflex areas in the hands are useful for the practitioner if for some reason the feet cannot be treated. This might occur if there was damage to a part of the foot or infection, in which case the foot would be treated in all the areas possible and the damaged or infected area treated through the corresponding area of the hand. Likewise, if a foot was injured entirely then the whole hand could be treated, remembering that the right hand corresponds to the right foot and the left hand corresponds to the left foot. In this latter case, treatment would therefore be given to one foot and one hand.

Self-treatment
Although reflexology is best given by a fully trained practitioner to obtain the maximum benefit from the treatment, it is a method which can be used to a certain extent for self-treatment. Reflexology is harmless, provided that it is applied correctly. The warnings which must be heeded are not to work too long and not to work too heavily. In the description of the various disorders which can be helped by reflexology other cautions have been mentioned, such as where there is a serious heart or circulatory disorder, diabetes or pregnancy. The tendency with self-treatment is to work on isolated reflex areas related to the condition requiring help but, while this may ease symptoms, the total balancing effect of the treatment will not be achieved. However, the relief of symptoms is obviously of benefit. Many people find the hands more useful for self-treatment than the feet since they are more easily reached and massage of reflex areas in the hands can be applied very conveniently at any time of the day and at any place without drawing attention to the fact that self-treatment is being applied. This can be done while, for example, watching television, waiting for a train or in a short break from work. For those who try self-treatment without success, do not disregard reflexology completely — it may well be that results could be obtained if a qualified practitioner was visited.

The use of various gadgets which claim to give reflexology treatment are not recommended — the hands are best used to apply massage to the reflex areas. It is also possible to buy sandals described as reflexology sandals and these should be viewed with some caution! With most makes of these sandals, the stimulation of the reflex areas, if achieved, is certainly not even and if they are worn for any length of time they could possibly overstimulate some areas and create an imbalanced situation. However, some people do find these types of shoe comfortable and if worn for short periods of time the stimulation received may well help the circulation in the feet and legs and give a slight toning up to the body with a feeling of more energy. Foot rollers are also available and, provided that they are made with smooth edges to them, they can be very useful in helping to improve the muscle tone of the feet and also the blood circulation in the feet. They can help to make the feet less stiff, a problem often found in the elderly, and can have an overall relaxing effect on the whole body. The rollers are not usually precise enough in their massage of the feet to be considered as giving reflexology treatment.

An awareness of the potential capabilities of reflexology does, in most cases, give people a much greater appreciation of their hands and, more particularly, their feet which are often a rather neglected part of the body. Caring for the hands and feet is a means of caring for the whole body, and massage to these areas as provided in reflexology treatment is not only valuable in helping correct ill-health but also in preventing ill-health. It helps the body to relax, so that tension and stress are reduced and can be coped with more easily.

Chapter 8

Finding a Reliable Reflexologist

Once the decision to try reflexology treatment has been taken, then the next important step is to try to find a good practitioner of the method. The recent growing interest in the alternative therapies has led to an increase in the number of people practising the various therapies and also an increase in the number of training courses available for them. This has its advantages and disadvantages and with reflexology there is much variation in the qualifications and proficiency of practitioners. In addition, in Britain at present there are no laws governing the practice of the alternative therapies, so there is nothing to stop an unqualified person setting up a practice for any of them, provided that they do not call themselves a doctor of medicine without having the appropriate medical qualification.

There are several training schools for reflexology, some of which teach to a higher standard than others. The first reflexology training school established in this country was started by the late Doreen E. Bayly who having run training courses since the early 1960s both in Britain and on the continent formed her own school in 1968 called the Bayly School of Reflexology. The School still runs regular training courses and students have to pass a written and practical test before being issued with a Certificate. The format for the courses has changed over the years and the tests for a Certificate were first introduced in 1980. A few other training schools make their students pass tests before issuing a Certificate, but some training schools just offer a Certificate of Attendance. It does, however, seem vital that students receive a sound training if they are to see patients on a professional basis.

The main training schools are able to give the names and addresses of trained practitioners in the various areas of the country and there is now a considerable number of people practising reflexology. Practitioners are allowed to advertise and names and addresses may be found in health magazines and sometimes in local newspapers. A local health shop will also probably be aware of the practitioners in their area. An advertisement does not necessarily mean that the person advertising is qualified, so it is most important that when contacting someone with a view to receiving treatment that they are asked where they trained and perhaps the length of their training — anyone properly qualified will not feel embarrassed to give this information. The other initial question must be about the cost involved for treatment, remembering that a course of treatment will probably be necessary. If an appointment is made, it is wise to look at the practitioner's Certificate at the first visit to make sure that they are genuine.

No elaborate equipment is required to give reflexology and so it not uncommon to find practitioners working from a room in their own home. A comfortable recliner-type chair should be used for the treatment and if this type of facility is not available then the treatment is not being approached in a very professional way. Many centres for alternative therapies have now been established around the country and it is usual for a reflexology practitioner to be included among the therapists working at such centres.

Reflexology and Other Therapies

Often reflexology is one treatment offered by an alternative therapist along with other therapies and this can sometimes be useful. It is important in these instances, though, that if reflexology treatment is offered that it is given in its full form with massage of all the areas of the feet and not just massage of a few areas. Some therapists may use reflexology as a means of diagnosis and then treat with other methods.

Since the treatment is harmless, provided it is applied correctly and certain precautions considered, it is possible to combine reflexology with other treatments. First, it will not interfere with any treatment being given by a doctor unless this involves certain drugs being taken and there is no harm done in telling the doctor that reflexology treatment is being tried. If acupuncture treatment is being followed there is probably little point in having reflexology treatment at the same time since the two are working in a similar manner on the body, but there are times when reflexology is of benefit when acupuncture is not and vice versa. The treatment can combine with osteopathy and some osteopaths may give reflexology treatment to relax a patient before manipulation. There will also be no contraindications if herbal medicine or homoeopathic remedies are being taken.

The effectiveness of reflexology treatment can sometimes be helped by other factors, the most important of which is probably diet. There are many conditions where the treatment cannot be 100 per cent effective unless alterations in diet are followed and it is not unusual for a practitioner to enquire as to the patient's diet and make some helpful suggestions. A diet sheet may well be issued at the first treatment, with a general guide to a wholesome healthy pattern of eating. Other helpful combinations with reflexology include the Bach Flower remedies, vitamins and minerals. The Bach Flower remedies are thirty-eight natural remedies all prepared from the flowers of wild plants, bushes and trees and which are used to treat the emotional state of a person rather than the physical conditions. They can be most helpful when there are negative states of mind present which may be preventing treatment from being fully effective. Vitamins and minerals can also be useful supplements to treatment, especially if the diet being followed is poor. Many people now take these supplements since they are readily available from health stores and chemists but the choice is almost too great. The practitioner will often be able to give advice on the use and necessity of such supplements.

In conclusion it is hoped that, having decided to try

reflexology treatment and having found a good practitioner, the results are successful. The treatment does not claim to be able to help everyone and every condition, but the majority of people will benefit. Reflexology must surely be one of the most pleasant treatments available — to lie back for nearly an hour and have all the reflex areas in the feet massaged is a relaxing, health-giving and wonderful experience.

Useful Addresses

UK

The British Reflexology Association (Secretary)
12 Pond Road
London SE3 9JL   Tel. 01-852 6062

The Bayly School of Reflexology
(the official teaching body of the British Reflexology
Association)
Monks Orchard
Whitbourne
Worcester WR6 5RB   Tel. Knightwick (0886) 21207

USA

New York School for Shiatsu and Reflexology
149E 81st Street
NYC, NY 10028

Reflexology/Ministry of Healing
3828 Kramer St
Harrisburg
PA 17109

Reflexology Workshop
1533 Shattuck
Berkeley
CA 94709

Index

In the same series ...

ACUPUNCTURE

A Patient's Guide

Dr Paul Marcus. A complete practical guide for the patient contemplating treatment by acupuncture. Uses western scientific explanations to describe acupuncture therapy in all its aspects in language a lay reader can easily understand. Dr Marcus, a medically trained practising acupuncturist, explains what a patient can expect from acupuncture and answers such questions as: Does acupuncture hurt? How does it work? What are the dangers? With an account of the history of acupuncture and a simple explanation of the facts so far known, it provides a refreshingly modern approach to a subject we all should know about. Contents include: which illnesses respond to acupuncture; how treatment is carried out; treatment with needles and moxibustion; the disadvantages and case histories.

HOMOEOPATHY

A Patient's Guide

Dr Anne Clover. An excellent introduction to the ideas basic to homoeopathy. Written in non-technical language, it describes homoeopathic prescribing, informs readers what to expect when being treated by a homoeopathic doctor, and answers such questions as: What is homoeopathy? How does it work? Is it safe? Can it be combined with other medicine? Dr Clover, a practising homoeopathic doctor, reviews the discoveries of Hahnemann — the founder of the homoeopathic system of medicine, and discusses why it is rapidly gaining in popularity.